Emergency
Care and Transportation of the Sick and Injured

Case Studies

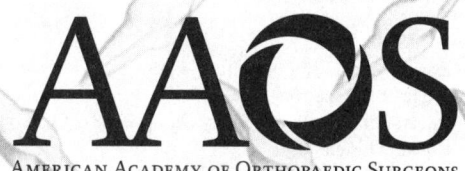
AMERICAN ACADEMY OF ORTHOPAEDIC SURGEONS

Series Editor:
Andrew N. Pollak, MD, FAAOS

Author:
Beth Ann McNeill, MS(c), EMT-B

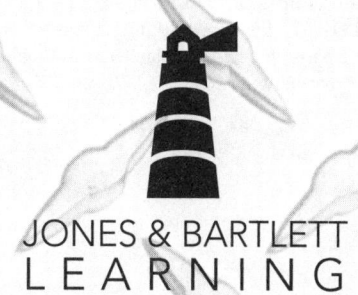
JONES & BARTLETT
LEARNING

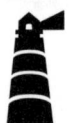 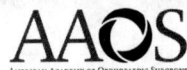

World Headquarters
Jones & Bartlett Learning
5 Wall Street
Burlington, MA 01803
978-443-5000
info@jblearning.com
www.jblearning.com

Chief Education Officer: Mark W. Wieting
Director, Department of Publications: Marilyn L. Fox, PhD
Managing Editor: Barbara A. Scotese
Associate Senior Editor: Gayle Murray

AAOS Board of Directors, 2011–2012

President: Daniel J. Berry, MD
First Vice-President: John R. Tongue, MD
Second Vice-President: Joshua J. Jacobs, MD
Past President: John J. Callaghan, MD
Treasurer: Frederick M. Azar, MD
Treasurer-elect (ex officio): Andrew N. Pollak, MD
Jeffrey O. Anglen, MD
William J. Best
Kevin P. Black, MD
Wilford K. Gibson, MD
Mininder S. Kocher, MD, MPH
Gregory A. Mencio, MD
Fred C. Redfern, MD
Steven D.K. Ross, MD
Naomi N. Shields, MD
David D. Teuscher, MD
Daniel W. White, MD, LTC, MC
Karen L. Hackett, FACHE, CAE *(ex officio)*

Jones & Bartlett Learning books and products are available through most bookstores and online booksellers. To contact Jones & Bartlett Learning directly, call 800-832-0034, fax 978-443-8000, or visit our website, www.jblearning.com.

Substantial discounts on bulk quantities of Jones & Bartlett Learning publications are available to corporations, professional associations, and other qualified organizations. For details and specific discount information, contact the special sales department at Jones & Bartlett Learning via the above contact information or send an email to specialsales@jblearning.com.

Copyright © 2013 by Jones & Bartlett Learning, LLC, an Ascend Learning Company

All rights reserved. No part of the material protected by this copyright may be reproduced or utilized in any form, electronic or mechanical, including photocopying, recording, or by any information storage and retrieval system, without written permission from the copyright owner.

The procedures and protocols in this book are based on the most current recommendations of responsible medical sources. The American Academy of Orthopaedic Surgeons and the publisher, however, make no guarantee as to, and assume no responsibility for, the correctness, sufficiency, or completeness of such information or recommendations. Other or additional safety measures may be required under particular circumstances.

This textbook is intended solely as a guide to the appropriate procedures to be employed when rendering emergency care to the sick and injured. It is not intended as a statement of the standards of care required in any particular situation, because circumstances and the patient's physical condition can vary widely from one emergency to another. Nor is it intended that this textbook shall in any way advise emergency personnel concerning legal authority to perform the activities or procedures discussed. Such local determination should be made only with the aid of legal counsel.

Additional photographic and illustration credits appear on page 251, which constitutes a continuation of the copyright page.

Production Credits

Chairman, Board of Directors: Clayton Jones
Chief Executive Officer: Ty Field
President: James Homer
SVP, Editor-in-Chief: Michael Johnson
SVP, Chief Operating Officer: Don Jones, Jr.
SVP, Chief Technology Officer: Dean Fossella
SVP, Chief Marketing Officer: Alison M. Pendergast
Executive Publisher: Kimberly Brophy
VP of Sales, Public Safety Group: Matthew Maniscalco
Executive Acquisitions Editor—EMS: Christine Emerton
Director of Sales, Public Safety Group: Patty Einstein
Senior Editorial Assistant: Amber Hodge
Production Manager: Jenny L. Corriveau
Associate Production Editor: Nora Menzi
Director of Marketing: Alisha Weisman
VP, Manufacturing and Inventory Control: Therese Connell
Text Design: Anne Spencer
Cover Design: Kristin E. Parker
Rights and Permissions Manager: Katherine Crighton
Photo Research Supervisor: Anna Genoese
Cover Image: Cover photographed by Ray Kemp/911 imaging <www.911imaging.com>. Special thanks to Susan Hertzler, Terrance Jackson, Cass Wilson, AllMed, St. Charles County, MO Ambulance District; Photo of EMT patch: © Stephen Coburn/ShutterStock, Inc.
Printing and Binding: Courier Corporation
Cover Printing: Courier Corporation

Some images in this book feature models. These models do not necessarily endorse, represent, or participate in the activities represented in the images.

Library of Congress Cataloging-in-Publication Data

Emergency care and transportation of the sick and injured case studies / American Academy of Orthopaedic Surgeons ; Beth A. McNeill.
    p. ; cm.
    Includes index.
    ISBN-13: 978-0-7637-8063-0 (pbk.)
    ISBN-10: 0-7637-8063-4 (pbk.)
    1. Medical emergencies—Case studies. 2. Transport of sick and wounded—Case studies. I. American Academy of Orthopaedic Surgeons. II. Title. [DNLM: 1. Emergency Treatment—Case Reports. 2. Emergency Treatment—Problems and Exercises. 3. Medical History Taking—Case Reports. 4. Medical History Taking—Problems and Exercises. 5. Moving and Lifting Patients—Case Reports. 6. Moving and Lifting Patients—Problems and Exercises. 7. Physical Examination—Case Reports. 8. Physical Examination—Problems and Exercises. 9. Transportation of Patients—Case Reports. 10. Transportation of Patients—Problems and Exercises. WB 18.2]
    RC86.7M318 2012
    616.02'5—dc22
                                                                                    2011004057
6048
Printed in the United States of America
15 14 13 12 11   10 9 8 7 6 5 4 3 2 1

Contents

CASE 1	Workforce Safety and Wellness	1
CASE 2	Medical, Legal, and Ethical Issues	7
CASE 3	Communication and Documentation	13
CASE 4	Patient Assessment	20
CASE 5	Airway Management	28
CASE 6	Shock	35
CASE 7	Respiratory Emergencies	45
CASE 8	Cardiovascular Emergencies	53
CASE 9	Neurologic Emergencies	62
CASE 10	Gastrointestinal and Urologic Emergencies	72
CASE 11	Endocrine and Hematologic Emergencies	80
CASE 12	Toxicology	87
CASE 13	Psychiatric Emergencies	94
CASE 14	Gynecologic Emergencies	100
CASE 15	Bleeding	109
CASE 16	Soft-Tissue Injuries	116
CASE 17	Face and Neck Injuries	123
CASE 18	Head and Spine Injuries	130
CASE 19	Chest Injuries	138
CASE 20	Abdominal and Genitourinary Injuries	145
CASE 21	Musculoskeletal Injuries	152
CASE 22	Environmental Emergencies	159
CASE 23	Obstetrics and Neonatal Care	167
CASE 24	Pediatric Emergencies	178
CASE 25	Geriatric Emergencies	184
CASE 26	Patients With Special Challenges	192
CASE 27	Lifting and Moving Patients	201
CASE 28	Transport Operations	210
CASE 29	Vehicle Extrication and Special Rescue	216
CASE 30	Incident Management	226
CASE 31	Terrorism Response and Disaster Management	236

Index 243
Photo Credits 251

Acknowledgments

The American Academy of Orthopaedic Surgeons, the authors, and Jones & Bartlett Learning wish to thank the following contributors and reviewers who were involved in the development of this resource.

■ Contributor

Christi Montellato, EMT-P
HeartShare Training Services Inc.
San Jose, California

■ Reviewers

George W. Contreras, MPH, MS, CEM, EMT-P
Associate Professor & Director of Allied Health Sciences
Kingsborough Community College, The City University of New York
Brooklyn, New York

Lieutenant Mark B. Fowler
Flagler County Fire Rescue
Bunnell, Florida

Randy L. Fugate, NREMTP, CCEMTP, PNCCT
NC Level II EMS Instructor/Coordinator
Critical Care Coordinator
Asheville Buncombe Technical Community College & Mission Health System Regional Transport Services
Asheville, North Carolina

Derek Hunt, NR/CCEMT-P, FP-C
ShandsCair, Shands at the University of Florida
Gainesville, Florida

Dean C. Meenach, RN, BSN, CEN, CCRN, CPEN, EMT-P
Director of EMS Education
Mineral Area College
Park Hills, Missouri

David Newberry, EMT-P
Dekalb Technical College
Clarkston, Georgia

Michael H. Wilhelm, BSN, RN, CCRN, CEN, AEMT-CC, CIC
West Queens Emergency Medical Training Institute
Floral Park, New York

■ From the Author

First and foremost I would like to thank my family and friends for their support in writing this book. My husband, Andy, and my daughters, Whitney and Clarissa, were real troopers and my biggest supporters when it came to my endless hours of writing and rewriting. Thank you to Rich Beebe for encouraging me to write an EMS book. A special thanks to Christine Emerton for supporting my idea and running with it. I am also grateful to my editor, Amber Hodge, for coming on board with this project and being so supportive of my creative ideas. Thank you to the following members of the Brighton Fire Department (NY) who provided information for this book: Firefighter Bruce Blackman for his advice on dog bites and Firefighter Steve "Snapper" Preston and Captain Scott Fitch for their input on firefighter rehab. Lastly, I would like to thank my students, past, present, and future, for giving me the opportunity to do what I love: teach.

■ Dedication

To my first partner in EMS, Marty Michael, who taught me so many tricks of the trade: I will remember you until the cows come home.

And to Tim Karnisky, who not only became my best friend, but also my brother. Tim exemplified loyalty and dedication and always had my back, in and out of EMS.

Gone but never forgotten.

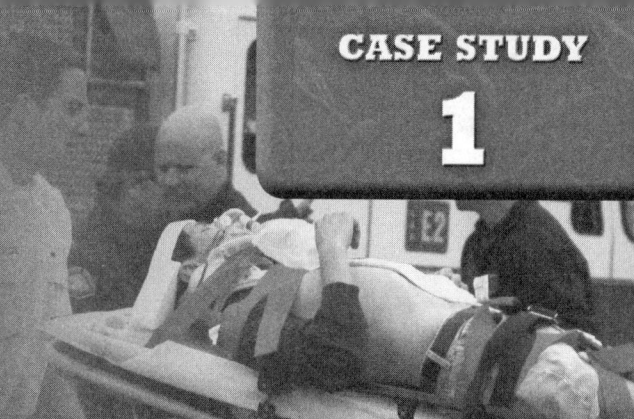

CASE STUDY 1

Workforce Safety and Wellness

Man Needing a Lift Assist

Just as you finish eating dinner with the crew, the tones sound, and your pager goes off. The call is for a 53-year-old man who needs a lift assist at 2721 Lamson Road. You are familiar with this location because you, your partner, and the other crews have responded there before. You recall that the man is overweight and a paraplegic. Your dispatcher confirms the call and alerts the emergency dispatcher that you will be en route momentarily, with no lights or sirens (priority 4). Time out is 1849.

Your partner, Ryan, begins to complain about this patient while en route to the call. He tells you that this patient has abused emergency medical services (EMS) and fire services for the past 10 years after he became a paraplegic as the result of a motor vehicle crash. You remind Ryan that responding to calls like this one is part of the job, even though it can be frustrating. The patient weighed approximately 300 pounds the last time you saw him, about 4 months ago, and you are concerned about being able to move the patient without calling for additional help.

You are greeted at the door by the patient's wife, Barbara, who explains that her husband, Floyd, slid off the toilet and landed on the floor. Barbara is frustrated that Floyd cannot help himself up and that she is unable to lift him alone. Floyd does have a patient lift; however, it is in need of repair and will not be fixed until tomorrow.

You enter the bathroom to find Floyd on the tile floor between the toilet and the shower stall. He is partially leaning against the wall for support. He has a look of frustration on his face, but manages to utter a greeting when you enter. You introduce yourself and he says, "Nothing hurts. I just want to get up off this floor."

Question 1

Prior to moving a patient, what question(s) would you ask the patient, spouse, or family member?

You assess Floyd's level of consciousness and determine that he is alert and oriented. He has no shirt on, just boxer shorts and socks. He has a patent airway, and he is breathing at a regular rate with no retractions. His skin is pale and cool to the touch. However, you recall that this is normal for Floyd because of his paralysis. You do not see any blood on the floor or bleeding from anywhere on the patient **Table 1**.

Barbara confirms that Floyd did not injure himself or lose consciousness when he slipped off of the toilet. She explains that she was coming in to assist him into his seat in the shower when he became impatient and wanted to try to move himself. His arms were too weak to hold his body weight and he slid to the floor. Floyd tells you that he is cold because he has been undressed for the past 20 minutes and that he simply wants help moving to his bedroom so that he can get dressed.

Workforce Safety and Wellness

Table 1 — Primary Assessment Findings for Floyd

General impression	53-year-old man in need of a lift assist.
Chief complaint	Unable to get up.
Level of consciousness	Alert and oriented to person, place, day, time, and event.
Airway	Open and patent.
Breathing	Regular rate with no retractions.
Circulation	Skin is pale and cool to the touch (normal for patient). Radial pulse on right side is strong and regular. No signs of bleeding.
Life threats	No apparent life threats; no trauma.
Pain	No pain.
Glasgow coma scale (GCS)	Score: 15 (eye opening, 4; verbal response, 5; motor response, 6).
Interventions	Assessment of vital signs.

Before you attempt to move Floyd, you obtain a full set of vital signs **Table 2**.

Table 2 — Baseline Vital Signs for Floyd

Respirations	16 breaths/min, full and regular
Pulse	88 beats/min, strong and regular
Skin	Cool, pale, and dry
Blood pressure	140/88 mm Hg
Oxygen saturation	99% on ambient air

Question 2

Which technique would you use to move the patient from the floor to the bedroom?

Question 3

What could be done to minimize the chances of dropping or injuring a bariatric patient during a move?

Now that you have determined that Floyd is only in need of a lift assist, you look at Ryan to see if he is thinking the same thing you are—you will probably need extra help moving this patient. You get your answer, but not the one that you were hoping for. Ryan tells you to grab Floyd's legs and he will lift from the top, under Floyd's armpits.

Question 4

Do you agree with your partner's decision to lift a bariatric patient without additional assistance? Why or why not?

You will only need to carry Floyd a few feet from the floor to the seat of the wheelchair. You wait for Ryan's count and lift his legs. As you do this you can see a grimace come across Ryan's face, which is now turning bright red. Before you have a chance to ask if Ryan is okay, Floyd is placed, rather abruptly, into his wheelchair. Ryan looks like he is in agony and can barely stand up. Floyd says that he is happy to be off the floor and uses the electronic controls on his wheelchair to move back toward the bedroom, with Barbara following close behind. Neither one of them notices that Ryan is doubled over in pain.

Question 5

What can be done to prevent an injury to yourself or a colleague while attempting to move a bariatric patient?

You follow Floyd and Barbara to the bedroom to obtain another set of vital signs **Table 3**. You also gather a SAMPLE history from Floyd and his wife, which includes his signs and symptoms, allergies, medications, pertinent past medical history, last oral intake, and the events leading up to the injury or illness **Table 4**. You have them sign a release before returning to Ryan.

Table 3 Second Set of Vital Signs for Floyd

Respirations	18 breaths/min and regular
Pulse	80 beats/min, strong and regular
Skin	Warm, pale, and dry
Blood pressure	138/90 mm Hg
Oxygen saturation	99% on ambient air

Table 4 SAMPLE History for Floyd

Signs and symptoms	Unable to get up off the floor.
Allergies	Penicillin.
Medications	Multivitamin, docusate (Colace), gabapentin, baclofen.
Pertinent past medical history	History of spinal cord injury, occasional bed sores.
Last oral intake	Lunch approximately 5 hours prior.
Events leading up to the injury or illness	Slid off toilet to floor while attempting to enter shower.

Ryan tells you that he injured his back during the lift and will need to call out of service for the rest of the shift. You assist him back to the rig and call your acting lieutenant to advise him of the situation.

Case Analysis

Question 1

Prior to moving a patient, what question(s) would you ask the patient, spouse, or family member?

It is important to ask patients about their immediate condition before they are moved so you do not aggravate an existing condition. Does anything hurt? Did the patient lose consciousness? Where does the patient need to be moved? In this case study, was the patient dizzy or light-headed before or after he slid off the toilet? Was any injury sustained? Is the patient able to assist with the move?

Question 2

Which technique would you use to move the patient from the floor to the bedroom?

Call for additional assistance if you feel you cannot move the patient with only the help of your partner. It is estimated that nearly 100 million adults in the United States are overweight or are obese. This translates to a larger obese or overweight patient population. Back injuries account for the largest number of missed days at work and both temporary and permanent disability. When preparing to move a patient, you should estimate the weight of the patient before attempting to move him. If using proper technique, it is reasonable to expect that you and your partner could safely lift and move a patient up to about 200 pounds. It is safer, however, to try to use four rescuers whenever your resources will allow. More than half of the weight of a patient is distributed near the head of the patient. With this in mind, the strongest partner should perform the lifting at the patient's head. With any lifting it is imperative to have good communication with your partner(s) and patient. It can be uncomfortable or even frightening for a patient being moved, especially when they do not know what to expect. One of the preferred methods of moving a patient from a seated or supine position, whom you do not suspect has suffered any potential extremity or spinal trauma, is to use the extremity lift. With the extremity lift, one EMT stands behind the patient, at his or her head, and has the patient cross his or her hands over his or her chest. The first EMT places one hand under each of the patient's armpits and then grasps the patient's wrists or forearms and pulls the torso up until the patient is in a seated or upright position. The second EMT moves to a position at the feet. As the EMT at the head gives the command, both stand fully upright and move the patient to the stretcher.

Question 3

What could be done to minimize the chances of dropping or injuring a bariatric patient during a move?

Good communication is paramount when moving any patient. Having a plan in place prior to the move is also key to moving patients safely.

Question 4

Do you agree with your partner's decision to lift a bariatric patient without additional assistance? Why or why not?

There are several lifting and moving principles to keep in mind before lifting a patient of any size and weight. Safety is an absolute first consideration in lifting and moving.

1. Size up the situation.
   - Estimate the patient's size and weight.
   - Determine which providers are available and assess their ability to lift.
   - Determine the limitations of the equipment you have available (eg, the maximum load capacity of the gurney/stretcher).
   - Know where you are moving your patient. Also, determine what obstacles might be in your way during egress.
   - How will you move this patient? What device will best suit this move?
2. Lifting and moving need to be executed in a coordinated manner. Each lift should be planned.
   - Communication with your partner(s) is key to a safe and successful move.
   - Communicate with the patient. Tell the patient what to expect. This includes setting rules for the move. For instance, have the patient keep his hands on his lap so he does not throw off your balance during the move. This will also prevent the patient's hands from being injured during the move.
3. Proper lifting techniques and good body mechanics need to be used on every move, regardless of whether your patient is obese. Best practices include, but are not limited to, the following:
   - Do not bend at the waist.
   - Flex at the hips when bending.
   - Use the large muscles of your legs to help with the lift.
   - Carry the weight close to your body.
   - Keep the weight evenly distributed.
   - Avoid overreaching or twisting during a lift.
   - Keep your back in line and in a locked position during the lift.
   - When using equipment (eg, gurney/stretcher), lift the device with your palms up because this position provides the greatest strength to your hands and arms during a lift.

It is imperative to use proper body mechanics any time you engage in lifting and moving a patient. When an overweight patient needs to be moved, call for additional assistance to ensure a careful, safe move.

Question 5

What can be done to prevent an injury to yourself or a colleague while attempting to move a bariatric patient?

The first step in preventing injury to the crew or patient is recognizing where a potential hazard exists. Knowing that a patient's weight is too much for two people to lift is the first clue to identifying probable risks. If your crew was familiar with this patient's size and weight from previous EMS encounters, then a call for assistance should have been made after being dispatched.

Patient Care Report for Floyd

EMS Patient Care Report				
Date: 09-09-2011	**Incident No.:** 011233	**Nature of Call:** Man fallen	**Location:** 2721 Lamson Road	
Dispatched: 1847	**En Route:** 1849	**At Scene:** 1855	**Transport:**	**At Hospital:**	**In Service:**

Patient Information	
Age: 53 **Sex:** Male **Weight (in kg [lb]):** 135 kg (300 lb)	**Allergies:** Penicillin **Medications:** Multivitamin, docusate (Colace), gabapentin, and baclofen **Past Medical History:** History of paraplegia for 10 years as a result of a motor vehicle crash (MVC) **Chief Complaint:** Unable to get up

Vital Signs				
Time: 1900	**BP:** 140/88	**Pulse:** 88 strong and regular	**Respirations:** 16 full and regular	**Spo$_2$:** 99%
Time: 1915	**BP:** 138/90	**Pulse:** 80 strong and regular	**Respirations:** 18 full and regular	**Spo$_2$:** 99%
Time:	**BP:**	**Pulse:**	**Respirations:**	**Spo$_2$:**

EMS Treatment (circle all that apply)

Oxygen @ 15 L/min via (circle one): NC NRM Bag-Mask Device	**Assisted Ventilation**	**Airway Adjunct**	**CPR**
Defibrillation	**Bleeding control**	**Bandaging**	**Splinting**	**(Other:)** Lift assist

Narrative

Dispatched to the residence of a man in need of a lift assist. Greeted at the door by the patient's wife and escorted into the bathroom to find the 53-year-old paraplegic man sitting upright on the floor in no apparent distress. Patient was found conscious, alert, and oriented to person, place, day, and time. Patient's skin was pale and cool to the touch, which is normal due to paraplegia. No signs of bleeding were noted. The patient's wife confirms that the patient did not injure himself when he fell. Patient denies losing consciousness and denies having any pain or injury. Patient requests to be lifted off the floor and taken to his bedroom where he can get dressed. Lifted patient under the arms and legs and placed him into his wheelchair. A second set of vital signs was assessed once the patient was in his wheelchair. Patient's vital signs were within normal limits, and his GCS score was 15. Patient signed the release form. Wife signed as a witness. Patient was advised to call 9-1-1 again if further assistance was needed. No further treatment provided. No transport. **End of report**

Case Study 2

Medical, Legal, and Ethical Issues

Man With Difficulty Breathing

You, Marty, and Julie have just finished breakfast at the base station on Sunday morning when a call comes in for a 67-year-old man with difficulty breathing. The address is 1223 Orchard Drive, a familiar residence to you and your crew. The patient has a history of chronic obstructive pulmonary disease (COPD) and frequently uses the ambulance service. Time out is 0959.

You arrive on scene at 1005 hours and are greeted on the front porch by Mrs. Lorie. "He's in the living room in his favorite chair again. Just can't seem to catch his breath today," she says, as she takes a slow drag from her cigarette.

You tell Mrs. Lorie, "We are going to need you to put out that cigarette because we are carrying oxygen and Mr. Lorie is on home oxygen." She grunts in disgust as she puts the cigarette out in an old soda can on the front porch.

Question 1

Are you under any obligation to enter this scene if you feel it is not safe?

As you enter through the front door, the smell of cigarette smoke fills the air. The oxygen tubing, snaking across the floor, is visible from the entryway. You follow it to the living room where you find Mr. Lorie sitting upright in his recliner. "Good morning, Mr. Lorie," Marty says.

Mr. Lorie replies, "Hi, guys. Back again, huh?" You see that Mr. Lorie has an open airway and his breathing, as usual, is labored. His nasal cannula is in place.

Just then, Mrs. Lorie walks into the room and says, "He needs to go to the hospital. He hasn't been feeling well all weekend."

Mr. Lorie yells, "Oh, Janice, be quiet! I am not going to the hospital this morning."

Question 2

How would you initially obtain consent from this patient?

"Mr. Lorie, can you tell us what is going on today and why you called for an ambulance?" you ask.

Mr. Lorie replies, "I didn't call, she did! I am fine. Nothing is different and I am not going to the hospital to sit around there all day."

Medical, Legal, and Ethical Issues

Question 3

Do patients have the right to refuse treatment and transport? Why or why not?

You respond, "Mr. Lorie, is it okay if we just check your vital signs and ask a few questions?" Mrs. Lorie cuts in, "He should go to the hospital! He can't even walk around the house today without being out of breath and saying he's dizzy."

Through a series of questions and answers, you determine that Mr. Lorie is alert and oriented to person, place, day, time, and event. Mr. Lorie denies losing consciousness, which is confirmed by his wife. You complete a primary assessment on Mr. Lorie **Table 1**.

Table 1 Primary Assessment Findings for Mr. Lorie

General impression	67-year-old man with difficulty breathing.
Chief complaint	Shortness of breath and dizziness.
Level of consciousness	Alert and oriented to person, place, day, time, and event.
Airway	Open and patent.
Breathing	Labored and shallow; home oxygen on via nasal cannula at 2 L/min. No trauma noted to chest.
Circulation	Upper extremity pulses are strong, rapid, and irregular. No visible bleeding. Skin is warm, dry, and gray.
Life threats	No apparent life threats; no trauma.
Glasgow coma scale (GCS)	Score: 15 (eye opening, 4; verbal response, 5; motor response, 6).
Interventions	Assessment of vital signs and patient history, and encourage patient to be transported.

Question 4

It seems clear to you that the patient has no interest in going to the hospital. What do you need to do before leaving the patient? What questions should you ask before the patient signs the release/refusal form?

Fortunately, Mr. Lorie allows you to assess his vital signs **Table 2** and obtain a SAMPLE history, including signs and symptoms, allergies, medications, pertinent past medical history, last oral intake, and events leading up to the illness or injury **Table 3**.

Table 2 — Baseline Vital Signs for Mr. Lorie

Respirations	24 breaths/min, shallow and labored
Pulse	98 beats/min and irregular
Skin temperature/condition	Warm, dry, and gray
Blood pressure	142/86 mm Hg
Oxygen saturation	95% on home oxygen

Table 3 — SAMPLE History for Mr. Lorie

Signs and symptoms	Shortness of breath due to history of COPD. Gray skin.
Allergies	Codeine, shellfish, and iodine.
Medications	Amoxicillin, furosemide, nebulized metaproterenol sulfate, mucodyne syrup, aspirin, propranolol, and budesonide metered-dose inhaler (MDI).
Pertinent past medical history	COPD, polycythemia, hypertension, and recent urinary tract infection.
Last oral intake	Bacon, eggs, toast, and coffee at 0730.
Events leading up to the illness or injury	Argument with wife increased shortness of breath. Wife called 9-1-1.

After assessing Mr. Lorie's vital signs and obtaining a history, you ask him again if he wants to go to the hospital. He emphatically declines, despite protests from his wife. You obtain a signed release from Mr. Lorie, and Mrs. Lorie signs as a witness. You advise Mr. Lorie to call 9-1-1 again if he feels worse. He says he will call his physician Monday morning for follow-up. You say goodbye and wish him a good day.

Question 5

How would you handle this situation?

Question 6

What is the best way to protect yourself from a potential lawsuit in a situation where a patient refuses care and/or transport?

Case Analysis

Question 1

Are you under any obligation to enter this scene if you feel it is not safe?

You are not under any obligation to enter a scene that is not safe or not secure. Scene safety is a priority. In this case, a lit cigarette could be considered potentially dangerous because you are carrying oxygen, which could accelerate combustion.

Question 2

How would you initially obtain consent from this patient?

Obtaining consent from a conscious patient begins with communicating with your patient. Saying "Hello" and telling him or her who you are and that you are there to help is a good place to start. Developing good rapport with your patients will always benefit the situation.

Question 3

Do patients have the right to refuse treatment and transport? Why or why not?

Competent adult patients have the right to refuse treatment and transport at any time. Keep in mind that calls that include patient refusal of treatment may lead to future litigation. Therefore, it is imperative that the emergency medical technician (EMT) assesses the patient's ability to make an informed decision. The EMT must ask the patient questions, assess the patient's answers, and observe the patient's behavior. This can be done by asking the patient where he or she is, what day of the week it is, and who is with the patient (family members, bystanders, etc.). The patient should clearly understand his or her situation and the possible repercussions for refusing care (ie, his or her condition could worsen, etc.). Encourage the patient to permit treatment and be transported. If the patient still refuses, be sure to explain what signs and symptoms to look for should the condition deteriorate. Always tell your patients that they may call 9-1-1 again should the need arise or they change their minds.

Question 4

It seems clear to you that this patient has no interest in going to the hospital. What do you need to do before leaving the patient? What questions should you ask before the patient signs the release/refusal form?

All mentally competent adults have the right to refuse treatment and/or transport. If the patient was forced into treatment and transport to the hospital, it could be viewed as kidnapping or imprisonment. As long as you have established that an adult patient is competent, he or she has a right to refuse care and transport. Document any assessment findings, the emergency care you provided, your efforts to obtain consent, and the responses to your efforts. Have the patient sign the release on your patient care report (PCR). You must also obtain a signature from a witness to the refusal. In this case, you could ask the patient's wife to sign as a witness. If family is not available to sign as a witness, you could ask a friend, coworker, or neighbor. Some law enforcement agencies will not sign as a witness on a PCR because it may be against their policy. You should check the standard operating guidelines with your local law enforcement agency for further clarification on this. Asking the patient if he fully understands what you have said and requiring the patient to repeat back to you his understanding of what has been said is imperative.

Question 5

How would you handle this situation?

There are several ways to handle this situation. First, it is important to remain calm and professional. Raising your voice or taking an aggressive posture may only serve to escalate the situation. Talk calmly to both the patient and family members. Explain to the patient's wife that you will assess her spouse, with his permission. You may also have to explain to her that you cannot force the patient to go to the hospital. You may suggest that your patient contact his physician as soon as possible to schedule an appointment. Reassure the patient and family that 9-1-1 can be called again to request service if the patient changes his mind.

Question 6

What is the best way to protect yourself from a potential lawsuit in a situation where a patient refuses care and/or transport?

In addition to a complete assessment, thorough documentation is key to preventing a lawsuit. It is crucial that this documentation be neat, detailed, and orderly. Write your documentation as if someone unfamiliar with the case needed to have an understanding of the whole story. Well-written documentation can prevent you from getting sued. Be sure to include in your documentation any pertinent negatives you found during the assessment. Pertinent negatives are findings that warrant no care or intervention. For example, if you asked the patient if he or she had any chest pain and he denied having any chest pain, this would be an example of a pertinent negative, and it could be documented this way: "Patient denied having any chest pain."

When you are writing the narrative portion of your PCR, be sure to use an organized approach. There are a few different ways this can be done. The subjective, objective, assessment, plan (SOAP) method; and the chief complaint, history and physical examination, assessment, treatment (Rx), and transport (CHART) method. Either of these methods can be useful in keeping your narrative organized, easy to read, and follow. These methods are explained in greater detail in the *Communication and Documentation* case study.

Patient Care Report for Mr. Lorie

EMS Patient Care Report (PCR)

Date: 04-14-11	Incident No.: 012341	Nature of Call: Difficulty breathing	Location: 1223 Orchard Drive	
Dispatched: 0957	En Route: 0959	At Scene: 1005	Transport:	At Hospital:	In Service: 1021

Patient Information

Age: 67 years **Sex:** Male **Weight (in kg [lb]):** 73 kg (162 lb)	**Allergies:** Codeine, shellfish, and iodine **Medications:** Amoxicillin, furosemide, nebulized metaproterenol sulfate, mucodyne syrup, aspirin, propranolol, and budesonide metered-dose inhaler (MDI) **Past Medical History:** COPD, polycythemia, hypertension (HTN), and recent urinary tract infection (UTI) **Chief Complaint:** Shortness of breath and dizziness

Vital Signs

Time: 1009	BP: 142/86	Pulse: 98 and irregular	Respirations: 24 shallow and labored	Spo$_2$: 95% on home oxygen
Time:	BP:	Pulse:	Respirations:	Spo$_2$:
Time:	BP:	Pulse:	Respirations:	Spo$_2$:

EMS Treatment
(circle all that apply)

Oxygen @ <u>15</u> L/min via (circle one): NC NRM Bag-Mask Device	Assisted Ventilation	Airway Adjunct	CPR
Defibrillation	Bleeding Control	Bandaging	Splinting	**(Other:)** Assessment of vital signs

Narrative

Dispatched to 1223 Orchard Drive for a 67-year-old man with difficulty breathing. Arrived on scene to be greeted by patient's wife. Found the patient seated in recliner in the living room. Patient denied any problems and stated that his wife unnecessarily called the ambulance. Patient denied needing or wanting any treatment or transport. Patient denied losing consciousness and this was confirmed by his wife. The patient's wife explained that her husband has had increased difficulty breathing and dizziness today, all of which the patient adamantly denied. The patient was found to be alert to person, place, day, time, and surroundings. He refused treatment interventions, but allowed us to perform a primary assessment, assess his vital signs, and obtain a history from him. Primary assessment revealed man with difficulty breathing, alert and oriented to person, place, day, time, and event. Airway open and free of obstructions; breathing is visibly shallow and labored with home oxygen in use via a nasal cannula at 2 L/min, no trauma to the chest; upper extremity pulses are strong, rapid, and irregular, no visible bleeding, and skin is warm, dry, and gray. Patient denied having chest pain, breathing difficulties, dizziness, and trauma. Patient last ate at approximately 0730 hours. Patient also refused transport to the hospital. Patient was advised of the potential health dangers if he did not seek medical care and his condition worsened. Advised patient to call 9-1-1 if condition changed or worsened. Also advised patient to call physician on Monday for follow-up care. Patient acknowledged his understanding of our concerns and assured crew that he would call 9-1-1 if his situation became worse. Patient signed medical release and his wife signed as a witness. No patient transport. **End of report**

CASE STUDY 3

Communication and Documentation

Man With Altered Mental Status in Police Custody

It is a cool fall evening. You and your partner, Sam, receive a call to the local police station for a 26-year-old man in a jail cell who needs treatment after being involved in an altercation at a bar. Time out from your quarters is 2217 hours. The call location is 2300 Elmwood Avenue.

You are greeted at the door of the station by Officer Austin and led to a holding cell where Patrick is in custody. You inquire about the incident on your way to the cell. You learn that the patient was involved in a fight with another man at a local bar about an hour ago. Both men were arrested for disorderly conduct. The police had requested emergency medical services response for Patrick because he was experiencing a headache, dizziness, and nausea. Officer Austin also informs you that Patrick's level of consciousness is decreasing and that his breathalyzer reading was 0.16 at 2110 hours.

As you approach the holding cell, you see that Patrick is seated on the bench with his head in his hands, moaning. You introduce yourself and tell Patrick that you are there to help. Patrick moans, "Okay," but does not look up. You ask your patient to state his name and he responds appropriately. Sam enters the holding cell and maintains manual cervical spine stabilization. You tell Patrick not to move his head. He has no idea what time it is, but you determine that Patrick is alert to person, place, and day of the week. You complete a primary assessment on Patrick Table 1.

Table 1	Primary Assessment Findings for Patrick
General impression	A 26-year-old man in police custody; involved in altercation, responsive and alert but moving slowly.
Chief complaint	Headache, dizziness, and nausea.
Level of consciousness	Alert to person, place, and day of the week. Responds when spoken to.
Airway	Intact, no visual obstructions, no fluids found.
Breathing	Breathing is shallow and equal bilaterally, no retractions noted. High-flow oxygen placed due to nausea and alleged decreasing level of consciousness. No deformities, contusions, abrasions, punctures, penetrations, paradoxical motion in the chest, burns, tenderness, lacerations, or swelling (DCAP-BTLS) noted to the chest.
Circulation	Upper extremity pulses are palpable, strong, and regular. Bleeding is not noted. Minor bruises noted on the forearms. Small bruise developing on forehead and left cheek.
Life threats	No apparent life threats.
Pain	9 on a scale of 1 to 10.
Pupils	Sluggish and equal to react.
Glasgow coma scale (GCS)	Score: 15 (eye opening, 4; verbal response, 5; motor response, 6).

You are able to gather a SAMPLE history of Patrick's signs and symptoms, allergies, medications, pertinent past medical history, last oral intake, and the events leading up to the illness or injury Table 2.

Table 2	SAMPLE History for Patrick
Signs and symptoms	Bruises to the left cheek, forehead, and both forearms. Patient reports nausea, dizziness, and a headache.
Allergies	Penicillin.
Medications	None, other than a seasonal flu shot in late September.
Pertinent past medical history	Nothing significant.
Last oral intake	Several pints of beer and some chicken wings at the bar.
Events leading up to the illness or injury	Patient was involved in a fight at the bar.

Patrick denies vomiting. He cannot remember if he received any trauma to the head during the fight, but he is certain that he was punched in the face and chest. Because of the mechanism of injury, unreliability of the patient history, and level of intoxication, you decide it is best to immobilize Patrick for treatment and transport.

Before you immobilize Patrick to the backboard you obtain a set of baseline vital signs and assess his pulse and motor and sensory function **Table 3**.

Table 3 — Baseline Vital Signs for Patrick

Respirations	18 breaths/min and shallow
Pulse	110 beats/min and strong
Skin	Pale, warm, and dry
Blood pressure	130/88 mm Hg
Oxygen saturation	96% on room air

Because Patrick is in police custody, Officer Austin accompanies you in the ambulance. Fortunately, you are only 10 minutes away from Strong Memorial Hospital. This gives you just enough time to complete your secondary assessment **Table 4**.

Table 4 — Secondary Assessment Findings on Patrick

Level of consciousness	Alert and oriented to person, place, and day of the week.
Airway	Intact and patent.
Breathing	No apparent breathing difficulties or distress. No breathing complaints.
Circulation	Pulses good in both upper extremities. Skin is warm, dry, and pale. No visible bleeding.
Head/neck	Patient has a headache. Bruising now noted to forehead and left cheek. Pupils are sluggish to respond. No other DCAP-BTLS noted on head or neck.
Chest	No DCAP-BTLS noted to chest. Lung sounds are clear and equal bilaterally with full expansion, although breathing is still somewhat shallow.
Abdomen	Soft, nontender, no rigidity.
Pelvis/genitalia	Intact, no pain on palpation/no priapism noted, no complaints of pain to the genitalia.
Lower extremities	No DCAP-BTLS or pain noted.
Upper extremities	Slight bruising to both forearms. Pulses good in both upper extremities. Skin is warm, dry, and pale.
Back	Unremarkable, no pain, no DCAP-BTLS.
Pain	Unable to rate at this time.
Glasgow coma scale (GCS)	Score: 15 (eye opening, 4; verbal response, 5; motor response, 6).

En route to Strong Memorial Hospital, Patrick starts to lose consciousness. He says he is feeling tired and wants to rest. You are preparing to complete another set of vital signs when your patient vomits. The vomit contains remnants of his dinner and smells like alcohol.

Sam pulls over and assists you in tilting the board to clear your patient's airway. Patrick is still semiconscious but complains that he doesn't feel well. Sam calls the hospital to let them know you are en route. Once you clear his airway, you assess his vital signs Table 5.

Table 5 Second Set of Vital Signs for Patrick	
Respirations	16 breaths/min and shallow
Pulse	100 beats/min and strong
Skin	Pale, moist, and cool
Blood pressure	138/86 mm Hg
Oxygen saturation	99% on oxygen

You give a report to the triage nurse, who tells you to take your patient to bed 2 in the trauma bay. You assist in transferring your patient to the emergency department staff. You give them a report and ask if they have any questions for you.

Question 1

What are some of the ways to organize the information in the patient care report (PCR)?

Question 2

Why is including pertinent negatives so important in documentation?

Case Analysis

■ **Question 1**

What are some of the ways to organize the information in the PCR?

There are a couple of ways to organize the information in a PCR. The important key to remember is to make sure your documentation is organized. One format that can be used is the SOAP format, which is a mnemonic device that stands for subjective, objective, assessment, and plan Table 6.

Table 6 The SOAP Format

Item	Description	Example
S–subjective	What you are told by the patient, family members, bystanders, first responders, or other witnesses on the scene.	Patient states, "My head hurts a lot" or bystander tells you, "He was hit in the face several times with a beer bottle."
O–objective	Your physical exam of the patient. Also includes signs that you see, hear, smell, measure, or otherwise assess with your senses.	Patient has bruising to both forearms found during the secondary assessment.
A–assessment	How you interpret the subjective and objective information you now have, in other words, a diagnosis of the patient's problem. The conditions you suspect and those you can rule out.	Patient appears to have sustained facial trauma and head trauma due to a fight at the local bar.
P–plan	Once you have determined what has happened to the patient, you need to document what you plan on doing for the patient and how you will treat what you found on assessment.	Cold therapy applied to forearms at site of bruising to help control swelling and pain. Patient placed in full cervical spine precautions.

Another charting method that may be used is the CHART method, which is a mnemonic device that stands for chief complaint, history and physical examination, assessment, treatment (Rx), and transport Table 7.

Table 7 — The CHART Format

Item	Description	Example
C–chief complaint	Patient's chief concern. Should be written in the patient's own words, whenever possible.	Patient states, "My head hurts a lot."
H–history and physical exam	This refers to the physical examination you have performed on your patient as well as the patient history, which includes: History of the present illness Nature of illness Mechanism of injury (MOI) Signs/symptoms, allergies, medications, pertinent past medical history, last oral intake, and events leading up to the illness or injury (SAMPLE) Onset, provocation, quality, radiation, severity, time of onset (OPQRST)	Patient has a no significant medical history. MOI is trauma to the head and face. Bruising now noted to forehead and left cheek.
A–assessment	Now that you have examined your patient, you will need to assess the patient's situation as a whole and determine your next course of action, which is the basis for the patient's treatment.	Patient will need to have cold therapy applied at bruising sites on forearms. Patient will also require spinal immobilization due to the MOI.
R–treatment (R_x)	What treatment will be given. This may include reassessing the patient en route to the hospital.	Patient placed on high-flow oxygen due to MOI, head trauma, nausea, and dizziness.
T–transport	To where the patient is transported to. This should only be to a facility or person with equal or higher training than you.	Patient transported to Strong Memorial Hospital to the trauma bay, bed 2. Registered nurse Goede, Dr. Kaplan, were present on transfer of patient.

Although many systems now use electronic documentation, it is still crucial to be thorough in your documentation, whether it is on paper or recorded electronically.

■ Question 2

Why is including pertinent negatives so important in documentation?

Pertinent negatives are negative findings that warrant no care or intervention. This information is important for good documentation because it shows that you thoroughly assessed the patient and ruled out potential problems.

Patient Care Report for Patrick

EMS Patient Care Report (PCR)

Date: 10-28-11	Incident No.: 20113258	Nature of Call: Injury due to altercation	Location: 2300 Elmwood Avenue		
Dispatched: 2216	En Route: 2217	At Scene: 2222	Transport: 2237	At Hospital: 2247	In Service: 2310

Patient Information

Age: 26 years
Sex: Male
Weight (in kg [lb]): 84 kg (185 lb)

Allergies: Penicillin
Medications: Seasonal flu shot in late September
Past Medical History: Nothing significant
Chief Complaint: Headache, dizziness, and nausea

Vital Signs

Time	BP	Pulse	Respirations	SpO$_2$
2227	130/88	110 and strong	18 and shallow	96% on room air
2242	138/86	100 and strong	16 and shallow	99% on oxygen

EMS Treatment (circle all that apply)

Oxygen @ **15** L/min via (circle one): NC **(NRM)** Bag-Mask Device | Assisted Ventilation | Airway Adjunct | CPR

Defibrillation | Bleeding Control | Bandaging | Splinting | **(Other:)** Suction

Narrative

Dispatched to police station at 2300 Elmwood Avenue for a patient in custody complaining of headache, dizziness, and nausea. Escorted to the holding cell by Officer Austin, where the patient is found seated holding his head in his hands. Patient was involved in a bar fight 1 hour prior. Patient was unaware of the current time but was aware of his surroundings, person, place, and the day of the week. Pulse and motor and sensory function were assessed before and after immobilization to the backboard and found to be positive in all four extremities both before and after immobilization. Patient's vital signs were assessed and then he was immobilized on a backboard due to the potential trauma from the mechanism of injury. Initial and secondary assessments were completed before arrival at the hospital. There were no apparent breathing difficulties or distress and pulses were good in both upper extremities. Bruising was noted to the forehead and both forearms, but no other signs of DCAP-BTLS were noted to the head, neck, chest, back, or upper or lower extremities. Patient's breathing was somewhat shallow but lung sounds were clear and equal bilaterally with full expansion. Administered high-flow oxygen, saturation at 99%. En route to the hospital, the patient dozed off and vomited. Driver stopped the ambulance en route to the hospital to assist the medic with suctioning. Suctioning was successful and there was no further vomiting. On arrival at Strong Memorial Hospital, we were greeted by the physician, nurse, and patient care technician. Full report given to hospital staff and patient was transferred to a trauma bed with the assistance of hospital staff. Patient was left in the care of hospital staff and the bed rails were left up and the bed lowered. **End of report**

CASE STUDY 4

Patient Assessment

Bicyclist Struck by Motor Vehicle

It is a warm, sunny afternoon and you are dispatched for a bicyclist struck by a car in the neighboring town of Pittsford. Your agency has a mutual aid agreement with Pittsford and they do not have an available crew. En route to the call, the dispatcher updates you that your patient is an 18-year-old woman who is conscious and on the side of the road. Police are en route to the scene as well. You and your partner, Andy, mark the time out to the call as 1445 hours.

Question 1

What are the steps involved in completing the scene size-up?

When you arrive, there is a county sheriff's deputy already on scene. Deputy Feehan tells you what happened as you walk toward the patient. Apparently, the woman did not look as she was crossing the street and was hit by a four-door sedan that was pulling out from a side avenue. The patient was not wearing a helmet.

Question 2

What steps are involved in performing the primary assessment?

Your patient is sitting upright on the grass about 15 feet from the roadway and the collision site. You introduce yourself to the patient, ask her to tell you her name, and tell her not to move her head as you gently hold cervical spine stabilization. She tells you her name is Whitney and she confirms that she is 18 years old. You determine that she is alert and oriented to person, place, day, and event. Her airway is intact and her breathing appears normal. Your partner provides high-flow oxygen by a nonrebreathing mask as a precaution while you perform the primary assessment **Table 1** and obtain baseline vital signs **Table 2**.

Table 1 — Primary Assessment Findings for Whitney

General impression	18-year-old woman, hit by car, sitting upright in grass, making eye contact, look of worry on her face.
Chief complaint	Pain to the forehead at injury site, some nausea.
Level of consciousness	Alert and oriented to person, place, day, time, and event.
Airway	Intact and patent.
Breathing	No apparent breathing difficulties or distress. No breathing complaints. Breathing is equal bilaterally.
Circulation	Pulses good in both upper extremities. Some bleeding noted to forehead at point of impact. Skin is warm, pale, and dry.
Life threats	Assess for possible head injury. No deformities, contusions, abrasions, punctures, penetrations, paradoxical motion in the chest, and burns, tenderness, lacerations, and swelling (DCAP-BTLS) to chest.
Pupils	Pupils are equal, round, regular in size, and react properly to light (PEARRL).
Pain	Forehead pain is 7 on a scale of 1 to 10.
Interventions	Cervical spine stabilization. Oxygen administration. Bleeding control.

Table 2 — Baseline Vital Signs for Whitney

Respirations	22 breaths/min and regular
Pulse	110 beats/min and regular
Skin	Warm, dry, and pale
Blood pressure	118/80 mm Hg
Oxygen saturation	98% on ambient air

Question 3

What is the purpose of history taking? What questions do you need to ask to obtain a thorough medical history?

You gather a SAMPLE history from Whitney, including signs and symptoms, allergies, medications, pertinent past medical history, last oral intake, and events leading up to the illness or injury **Table 3**.

Patient Assessment

Table 3 SAMPLE History for Whitney

Signs and symptoms	Abrasions noted to both palms, left knee, and left lower leg. Swelling noted to left knee. Bruising noted to forehead at injury site.
	Patient reporting a headache, pain to forehead at the injury site, and soreness to the upper back.
Allergies	Dairy and seasonal (pollen, mold).
Medications	Diphenhydramine (Benadryl), as needed.
Pertinent past medical history	No medical history other than the seasonal allergies. Healthy and athletic.
Last oral intake	Eggs, toast, and milk around 9:30 a.m.
Events leading up to the injury or illness	Patient was riding her bike across the intersection when she was struck by a car. Patient did not lose consciousness.

Question 4

On the basis of your primary assessment findings, how would you prioritize the care and transport of this patient?

Deputy Feehan tells you that Whitney's mother is on the way with an estimated time of arrival of approximately 10 minutes. You tell Whitney that there is a possibility that she may have injured her head and neck and because of that, you will need to place a collar and immobilize her to a backboard to get her moved to the ambulance. She says she understands but begins to cry, "My mom and dad are going to kill me! I didn't have my helmet on and they're going to be so upset!"

You apply a cervical collar, secure to the backboard, and place her in the back of the ambulance. Jennifer, a paramedic from a neighboring quadrant, arrives at the scene. As Jennifer boards the ambulance, you give her a report of your assessment findings.

Question 5

What is your role as a basic life support (BLS) provider now that an advanced life support (ALS) provider has arrived?

Whitney's mom arrives on the scene and Deputy Feehan asks if you could step out to speak to her. You leave Whitney in the care of the paramedic and step out to update the patient's mother.

Question 6

What verbal defusing strategies (method of communication) could you use when you are communicating with the patient's mother to ensure a calm situation?

After speaking with Whitney's mother, you allow her in the ambulance to see her daughter. Although they are a little emotional, they both remain calm when they see each other. You ask Whitney's mother to follow you to the hospital in her car, and you perform a more detailed assessment en route **Table 4**.

Question 7

What are the steps involved in the secondary assessment?

Table 4   **Secondary Assessment Findings for Whitney**

Level of consciousness	Remains alert and oriented to person, place, day, and event.
Airway	Still intact and patent.
Breathing	Rate is still within normal limits, no difficulty breathing, no pain on inspiration.
Circulation	Strong, regular pulses present in both upper extremities. No major bleeding noted. Skin is warm, pale, and dry.
Head/neck	Patient is reporting a headache and pain to the injury site on the forehead. Bruising now noted to the forehead. No other DCAP-BTLS noted on head or neck.
Chest	No DCAP-BTLS noted to chest. Lung sounds are clear and equal bilaterally with shallow expansion.
Abdomen	Soft, nontender, no rigidity.
Pelvis/genitalia	Pelvis is intact, no deformities or pain on palpation. Patient denies pain to genitalia region, inspection is deferred.
Lower extremities	Abrasion and slight swelling noted to left knee and lower leg. Pulse, movement, and sensation present in both lower extremities. No injuries noted to right lower extremity.
Upper extremities	Abrasions noted to both palms. Pulse, movement, and sensation present in both upper extremities. No other DCAP-BTLS noted in upper extremities.
Back/neck	Patient now reports soreness to her upper back due to the trauma of landing on the ground. There was no visible injury in the initial assessment.
Pertinent negatives	Patient denies loss of consciousness, denies difficulty breathing, and denies any neck or chest pain.
Pain	Patient rates her head pain as 8 on a scale of 1 to 10; her back pain is 6 out of 10; her knee pain is 5 out of 10.
Glasgow coma scale (GCS)	Score: 15 (eye opening, 4; verbal response, 5; motor response, 6).

Question 8

As you are transporting the patient to the hospital, what steps should be included in your reassessment?

Case Analysis

■ **Question 1**

What are the steps involved in completing the scene size-up?

The scene size-up is the first component to the patient assessment. This critical step will help to ensure your safety and the safety of your crew members while on a call. The scene size-up actually starts with the dispatch information. What information do you know before you go? Are there any updates given en route to the call? Are you aware of any specific scene hazards before you arrive at the call location? Prepare for the call by donning personal protective equipment (PPE). Always proceed to the call with caution and be aware of your surroundings. Look for hazards such as trees down, electrical wires down, hazardous materials that may have spilled or been discharged, animals that may pose a threat, dark houses, blocked entryways, or other hazards. It is also important to remember that scene safety is not a one-time job but rather a principle that should be maintained constantly throughout a call.

■ **Question 2**

What steps are involved in performing the primary assessment?

After the scene size-up, and after evaluating scene safety, the steps of the primary assessment are as follows:

- **General impression.** Begin your primary assessment by forming a general impression of the patient. The general impression is formed to determine the priority of the case and is based on your immediate assessment of the patient.
- Identify any life threats to the patient:
    - **Assess level of consciousness.** To determine the level of consciousness, talk to the patient and ask a few questions to determine responsiveness. Is the patient alert to person, place, time of day, and event?
    - **Assess airway.** Ask yourself these types of questions when assessing a patient's airway: Is the airway open? Will it stay open? What do I need to do to manage this airway? Does the airway need to be suctioned?
    - **Assess breathing.** Ask yourself these questions when assessing a patient's breathing: Is the breathing labored, shallow, or full? Is there difficulty breathing? Does the chest have equal expansion? Does the patient require supplemental oxygen? Does the chest have any obvious wounds that may impede breathing (such as deformities, contusions, abrasions, punctures, burns, lacerations, or swelling)?
    - **Assess circulation.** Ask yourself these questions when assessing a patient's circulation: Does the patient have full radial pulses? Is there bleeding anywhere on the body? What is the condition of the skin?
- **Begin lifesaving interventions if needed.** Any life threats that are found during the primary assessment need to be addressed immediately. For example, if you discover, during your assessment of breathing, that your patient has a hole in the chest (also known as a sucking chest wound), this wound would need to be immediately cared for and treated when it is found.
- **Perform a rapid scan.** A rapid scan should be performed prior to moving a patient to a longboard to determine if there are any other injuries that need to be managed before moving the patient. For example, if the patient has an angulated long bone fracture,

this would require stabilization before moving them to a longboard for transport. This rapid scan should only take 60–90 seconds to perform.
- **Determine priority of patient care and transport.** Does the patient need a trauma center? A burn center? Does the patient need urgent transport to the hospital or non-urgent transport?

Question 3

What is the purpose of history taking? What questions do you need to ask to obtain a thorough medical history?

The purpose of obtaining a complete patient history is to ensure that the provider finds less than obvious conditions with the patient. For example, it would be important to know if the patient lost consciousness or not during the injury. This information may very well help drive the direction of care that you take. A SAMPLE history is a must for all patients. Depending on the specific situation, you may have to ask more detailed questions. Document the following information:
- SAMPLE history: Signs/symptoms, allergies, medications, pertinent past medical history, last oral intake, and events leading up to the illness or injury.
- OPQRST for pain: Onset, provocation or palliation, quality, radiation, severity, and timing.
- Ask the patient to tell you the severity of pain based on the pain scale (1 through 10, with 10 being the worst pain ever felt).

In this case, the patient's mother has shown up to the scene. This would be a good opportunity to ask her about her daughter's medical history. You should ask if Whitney has any pertinent medical history, such as seizures or diabetes. Ask whether Whitney is current with her vaccinations.

Question 4

On the basis of your primary assessment findings, how would you prioritize care and transport of this patient?

Although this patient's vital signs are within normal limits for her age, the MOI is severe; transport to a trauma facility is necessary.

Question 5

What is your role as a BLS provider now that an ALS provider has arrived?

Your role as a BLS provider should remain just that: provide basic life-supporting care to the patient. There is a common misconception about the role of BLS providers in the presence of ALS care on scene. Oftentimes, EMTs retreat from patient care, thinking that their job has ended once ALS assistance has arrived. Nothing could be further from the truth. Good BLS care and assessment should continue while working in concert with ALS responders to achieve the ultimate goal of providing excellent patient care.

Question 6

What verbal defusing strategies (method of communication) could you use when you are communicating with the patient's mother to ensure a calm situation?

Verbal diffusing strategies are methods of communication used to help reduce stress, tension, or anger in patient contact situations. Speaking in a calm and reassuring voice and manner is the best approach to use when dealing with family, friends, or other relatives of the involved patient. Be direct, honest, and professional while showing that you genuinely care for the patient. Show that you are listening to the person talking by rephrasing what they say to you. Remember that nothing speaks louder than body language. How you carry yourself in public and on calls speaks volumes. Show that you are a team leader, in charge, and caring. A gentle, appropriate touch can be very reassuring. It is also best to adjust the way you speak to patients, family, and bystanders based on the age of the patient, stage of development, whether or not they have special needs, and keeping in mind cultural differences.

■ Question 7

What are the steps involved in the secondary assessment?

The secondary assessment involves a thorough head-to-toe exam.
- Assess vital signs using the appropriate monitoring devices: pulse, respirations, blood pressure, pupil response, oxygen saturation using pulse oximetry, and skin signs (color, temperature, and moisture).
- Perform a full body scan. Does anything look different now than it did during the initial assessment?
- Assess the respiratory system including airway patency and breathing rate, quality, depth, and lung sounds.
- Assess the cardiovascular system, including central and peripheral pulses, scarring to the chest or trauma, capillary refill time, and blood pressure.
- Assess the neurologic system by obtaining a GCS score and assessing motor and sensory function in all four extremities.
- Assess the musculoskeletal system, checking for DCAP-BTLS and assess pulse, motor function, and sensory function.
- Assess all anatomic regions. Use an organized approach, usually starting at the head, neck, and cervical spine, moving to the chest, and then to the abdomen, pelvis, and lower extremities, checking for DCAP-BTLS.

■ Question 8

As you are transporting the patient to the hospital, what steps should be included in your reassessment?

The purpose of reassessment is to check on any changes in patient status. Has the patient's condition improved or gotten worse or stayed about the same? Are there new signs and symptoms that were not evident before? Are your interventions working? Is the patient still alert and oriented? The steps to the reassessment strategy are as follows:
- Repeat the primary assessment
- Reassess vital signs
- Recheck interventions (eg, if oxygen was utilized, is the tank empty? If a splint was applied, does the patient still have pulses, movement, and sensation to that splinted extremity?)
- Identify and adjust your treatment based on changes in the patient's condition

Patient Care Report for Whitney

EMS Patient Care Report (PCR)

Date: 05-28-11	Incident No.: 2011345	Nature of Call: Bicyclist struck		Location: East Avenue and French Road, Pittsford	
Dispatched: 1444	En Route: 1445	At Scene: 1450	Transport: 1501	At Hospital: 1517	In Service: 1545

Patient Information

Age: 18 years	Allergies: Dairy and seasonal (pollen, mold)
Sex: Female	Medications: Diphenhydramine (Benadryl), as needed
Weight (in kg [lb]): 64 kg (140 lb)	Past Medical History: Seasonal allergies
	Chief Complaint: Pain to forehead and nausea

Vital Signs

Time	BP	Pulse	Respirations	SpO$_2$
1454	118/80	110 and regular	22 and regular	98% on ambient air
1506	120/80	100 and regular	20 and regular	100% on high-flow oxygen

EMS Treatment (circle all that apply)

Oxygen @ **15** L/min via (circle one): NC **(NRM)** Bag-Mask Device	Assisted Ventilation	Airway Adjunct	CPR
Defibrillation	**(Bleeding control)**	**(Bandaging to forehead)** **(Splinting lower left leg)**	**(Other:)** Spinal immobilization

Narrative

Dispatched to a call for an 18-year-old female bicyclist hit by a car. On arrival, we were greeted by Deputy Feehan from the sheriff's department. Patient found sitting upright on the side of the road. Patient was noted as being alert and oriented to person, place, day, time, and surroundings. Cervical spine stabilization was performed immediately. Patient was not wearing a helmet at the time of the injury. The patient denied losing consciousness and this was confirmed by a witness. Oxygen was administered due to the MOI and possible head injury. Patient's airway was intact and patent. The patient had no breathing complaints, and breathing was recorded as equal bilaterally. Pulses were noted as strong and regular in both upper extremities. Slight bleeding was noted to the forehead at the point of impact. After the primary assessment was completed, a cervical collar was applied and patient placed on a backboard. Sterile bandages and cold therapy were applied to an abrasion on forehead to control bleeding and lessen bruising. Patient's mother arrived on the scene and followed us to the hospital. A secondary assessment was completed en route to the hospital. The patient remained alert and oriented throughout transport. The patient's airway remained intact; breathing was within normal limits with no difficulty breathing reported and no pain to the chest area reported. No DCAP-BTLS noted to the chest, head, neck, except for the injury to the forehead. Pulses, movement, and sensation were present and strong in all four extremities. Skin was noted as warm, pale, and dry. The patient continued to report a headache and pain at the injury site. Lung sounds were clear and equal bilaterally with shallow expansion. Abdomen was noted as soft and nontender. The pelvis was noted to be intact with no deformities or pain noted. Abrasion and slight swelling noted to the left knee, lower left leg, and on both palms, but no other injuries noted otherwise on the extremities. Patient reported soreness of the back, but no visible injuries were noted prior to the patient being placed on the backboard. GCS score of 15 was obtained. Patient was talkative en route to the hospital with no further complaints. On arrival at the hospital, the patient was transferred to a registered nurse at the emergency department. **End of report**

CASE STUDY 5

Airway Management

Man With Congestive Heart Failure and Difficulty Breathing

It is Christmas night and you are dispatched for a 77-year-old man who has a history of congestive heart failure (CHF). Dispatch advises that the patient is experiencing difficulty breathing. After acknowledging the call at 135 Sycamore Street, you and your driver, Loreisha, head out to the ambulance in the engine bay. Time out for the call is 2056. Loreisha calls the dispatcher back to ask which advanced life support (ALS) unit will be coming to this call. "Medic 21 from Clinton and Broad," replies the dispatcher.

A young man anxiously greets you at the front door and tells you that his father is in the back bedroom. As you and Loreisha head down the hallway toward the bedroom, you catch a faint odor of urine in the air. You do not see any animals in the house and believe the odor may be coming from the bedroom. Just before you get to the doorway, you can hear a person's labored breathing. His son is close behind you telling you his father has a history of CHF and has not been feeling well for the past 2 or 3 days.

Question 1

Before you meet your patient, what clues tell you that your patient may be in a compromised medical condition?

Your patient, Mr. Donnelly, is sitting in the tripod position, his eyes pleading for help. You introduce yourself. "Hello. I am Bill and this is my partner Loreisha. We're here to help." Mr. Donnelly musters a faint smile. You notice that his head bobs with each breath despite the fact that he is receiving home oxygen. Through the unbuttoned, flannel pajama top, you can see that he is using accessory muscles to breathe and that he is sweating profusely. You also notice a scar lengthwise over his sternum.

Question 2

What do you think would be the best equipment to use to move this patient from his bedroom to the ambulance? In which position should you transfer this patient?

Loreisha leaves to get the stair chair and more blankets. You both realize that this patient will need to be moved quickly to the ambulance for further assessment and treatment, but you first perform a primary assessment **Table 1** and obtain a set of baseline vital signs **Table 2**.

Table 1. Primary Assessment Findings for Mr. Donnelly

General impression	77-year-old man with severe difficulty breathing.
Chief complaint	Difficulty breathing.
Level of consciousness	Alert and oriented to person, place, day, and event.
Airway	Open.
Breathing	Respiratory failure.
	Retractions around the clavicles and intercostal muscles, indicating accessory muscle use.
	Unable to speak in full sentences (one-to-two-word dyspnea).
Circulation	Weak, rapid pulses present in both upper extremities.
Life threats	Airway and breathing compromise.
Pertinent negatives	Patient and son deny loss of consciousness. Patient denies any pain but does have significant difficulty breathing.
	Patient's son denies any trauma to patient.
Pupils	Sluggish and irregularly shaped bilaterally.
Pain	Not identified.
Glasgow coma scale (GCS)	Score: 15 (eye opening, 4; verbal response, 5; motor response, 6).
Interventions	Airway management.
	Comfortably position the patient for transport.
	High-flow oxygen via a nonrebreathing mask.

Table 2. Baseline Vital Signs for Mr. Donnelly

Respirations	36 breaths/min, shallow and labored
Pulse	120 beats/min, regular and weak
Skin	Warm, moist, and pale in the face; cyanotic in the hands
Blood pressure	162/96 mm Hg
Oxygen saturation	88% on home oxygen at 4 L/min

You obtain a SAMPLE history from the patient's son, including signs and symptoms, allergies, medications, pertinent past medical history, last oral intake, and events leading up to the injury or illness **Table 3**.

Table 3	SAMPLE History for Mr. Donnelly
Signs and symptoms	Accessory muscle use; one-to-two-word dyspnea; cyanotic fingers; pale, moist skin; shallow and labored breathing.
Allergies	Morphine and latex.
Medications	Daily vitamins, furosemide (Lasix), polycarbophil (Fibercon), warfarin (Coumadin), diclofenac (Voltaren ophthalmic), and hydroxyzine (Atarax).
Pertinent past medical history	Triple bypass surgery 12 years ago, congestive heart failure, cataract surgery 3 weeks ago, hypertension, occasional constipation.
Last oral intake	Lunch approximately 6 hours prior to call. Did not feel up to eating dinner, according to the son.
Events leading up to the illness or injury	Ambulating with walker from bathroom to bedroom when shortness of breath occurred.

Loreisha returns with the stair chair and extra blankets. She tells you that the paramedics may be delayed in arrival because they are held up at a railroad crossing.

You and Loreisha move Mr. Donnelly to the stair chair in preparation to bring him out of the house and to the gurney. Mr. Donnelly is cooperative but still unable to speak in full sentences. He continues to nod or shake his head when you ask him questions. After covering the patient and checking the oxygen therapy, you wheel Mr. Donnelly to the front door and transfer him to the gurney.

Mr. Donnelly's son will meet you at Sheridan Community Hospital. On inquiry, you are told that the patient does not have a do not resuscitate order.

Question 3

What concerns do you have for maintaining this patient's condition en route to the hospital?

Despite the oxygen therapy, Mr. Donnelly's breathing remains labored and difficult. Mr. Donnelly is still unable to speak to you in full sentences and his skin color has not changed. Loreisha tells you that ALS is still about 15 minutes away. You ask her to request another medic from your agency to assist you with managing this patient and tell her to head to the hospital using lights and sirens.

Question 4

What treatment should you administer to assist your patient's decreasing respiratory effort? What could happen if you do not assist ventilation?

Question 5

What are potential airway management challenges for this patient?

Question 6

How might you best communicate with your patient about assisting with ventilation?

In the ambulance, you attach the bag-mask device to the on-board oxygen and set it at 15 L/min. You take a nasopharyngeal airway (NPA) out of the cabinet, and check the size to ensure it is correct for your patient. After lubricating the NPA, you explain to Mr. Donnelly, "I need to insert this small tube in your right nostril to help get air into your lungs." Although Mr. Donnelly's eyes are open, he does not give a response. He is completely exhausted. After sufficiently lubricating the airway adjunct, you gently insert the NPA into his right nostril. Fortunately, you do not meet any resistance. You place the bag-mask device on Mr. Donnelly's face and talk to him as you assist his ventilations. You tell him, "I am going to help you breathe now. I know you are very tired. Just breathe in as I squeeze the bag, Mr. Donnelly—breathe, breathe, breathe. You're doing great."

Loreisha tells you that Scott, another EMT from your agency, will be arriving soon to help manage this patient. There is still no word on when ALS will arrive.

Once Scott is on board and assisting with airway maintenance, you perform an abbreviated secondary assessment Table 4.

Table 4 Secondary Assessment Findings for Mr. Donnelly

Level of consciousness	Responds to questions with a nod of his head. Too difficult to speak due to respiratory failure and assisted ventilations.
Airway	Secured with an NPA and positioning.
Breathing	Assisted ventilations at 15 L/min.
Circulation	Pulses present in both upper extremities, weak and regular. Skin is cool, pale, and moist.
Head/neck	Deferred.
Chest	Equal expansion with assisted ventilations. Scar noted to chest from previous cardiac surgery.
Abdomen	Deferred.
Pelvis/genitalia	Deferred.
Lower extremities	Deferred.
Upper extremities	Deferred.
Back/neck	Deferred.
Pain	Patient denied pain.
Glasgow coma scale (GCS)	Score: 11 (eye opening, 4; verbal response, 1; motor response, 6).

Loreisha informs you that your estimated time of arrival to Sheridan Community Hospital is 6 to 8 minutes. Mr. Donnelly is still conscious. You take over maintaining the mask-seal for Scott as he squeezes the bag. Loreisha calls in to the hospital to inform them of the incoming patient.

Once at the hospital, the staff is waiting for you at the emergency entrance. Scott and Loreisha move the gurney as you continue to assist ventilations. The staff helps to transfer the patient and you give your report to the attending physician. Although you know Mr. Donnelly is a very sick man, you are glad that you have brought him to the hospital still conscious. You and your team have prevented him from going into full respiratory arrest and possibly cardiac arrest. As you all gather your equipment and head to the sinks to wash up, you see Mr. Donnelly's son. Loreisha tells him that his father is still conscious and shows him to the appropriate patient room.

Case Analysis

■ Question 1

Before you meet your patient, what clues tell you that your patient may be in a compromised medical condition?

Labored breathing is certainly one indicator of his compromised medical condition. It is not unusual to hear patients in respiratory distress laboring to breathe. They may be gasping for air (air hunger). Their lungs may be filled with fluid, so the breaths may sound wet when you hear them. The odor of urine in the home suggests incontinence, which can happen for a variety of reasons. This patient could be incontinent normally or acutely. His failing efforts to breathe may have frightened him to the point where he lost bladder control. A history of CHF is also an indicator of a poor medical state.

■ Question 2

What do you think would be the best equipment to use to move this patient from the bedroom to the ambulance? In which position should you transfer this patient?

A stair chair would be the best device to use. Some providers might bring a gurney into a home, although it is not generally advised due to the weight of the gurney itself and the lack of maneuverability in tight spaces. A stair chair will ensure that the patient remains in an upright or semi-upright position until you reach the gurney and the ambulance. Because of the patient's level of respiratory failure, this patient should be transported in an upright position. If the patient becomes unresponsive or is unable to maintain a patent airway, it is acceptable to lay the patient down to provide ventilations.

■ Question 3

What concerns do you have for maintaining this patient's condition en route to the hospital?

This patient will require aggressive airway management. Assisted ventilations, high-flow oxygen, and an airway adjunct will be needed. It is imperative to continue to talk to your patient and coach the breathing if he is still conscious during assisted ventilations. If ALS has not been called, be sure to request them for a call like this.

■ Question 4

What treatment should you administer to assist your patient's decreasing respiratory effort? What could happen if you do not assist ventilation?

The patient is not breathing adequately, as indicated by the signs and symptoms of respiratory failure, which include the following:

- The inability to speak in full or complete sentences
- Accessory muscle use
- Cyanosis
- Shallow breathing
- Rapid or slow breathing

When a patient is in this level of distress, immediate action is required on your part. This patient is not able to sustain proper oxygenation of his cells. It is imperative that you rapidly recognize this level of distress and act accordingly in assisting his breathing. One way to help the patient is to assist ventilation with a bag-mask device. Because the patient is still conscious, you need to talk to him and explain what you are doing. The mask will be placed over Mr. Donnelly's mouth and nose. Initially, you will squeeze the bag each time the patient inhales. After the first 5 to 10 ventilations are delivered, slowly begin to adjust the rate at which you deliver the ventilation. If Mr. Donnelly is breathing too rapidly, coach or talk him down to a slower rate, at the same time ventilating at a slower rate. If he is breathing too slowly, coach him to a faster rate while ventilating at a faster rate.

Proper technique is crucial to prevent gastric distention when assisting ventilations. Gastric distention occurs when too much air enters the stomach instead of the lungs and can oftentimes lead to vomiting. Vomit can then enter the trachea and cause an airway obstruction. Gastric distention may occur because the ventilations are too forceful or too rapid. Maintain a good mask seal and be sure to watch for chest rise *and* fall during ventilation.

The second option for assisting a patient in respiratory distress or failure is to use continuous positive airway pressure (CPAP). Many people diagnosed with sleep apnea, a lack of spontaneous breathing during sleep, currently use CPAP. It has been proven to be quite effective. CPAP has also been added to the prehospital environment as a means of providing ventilator assistance. CPAP assists in increasing pressure in the lungs and opening collapsed alveoli. The machine uses oxygen to force or deliver positive pressure into the airway and lungs. Although CPAP is widely used in the United States in the prehospital environment at the EMT level, be sure to check with your local protocols for use in your area.

If you do not assist the patient's respirations, the patient may end up in respiratory arrest and his condition could quite possibly spiral into cardiac arrest.

Question 5

What are potential airway management challenges with this patient?

Many airway management challenges may be present during respiratory failure in a patient with CHF. Keeping the patient's airway clear of secretions as well as successfully keeping track of his breathing will require constant monitoring and mastery of proper ventilation techniques. Be prepared to suction the airway as needed and continuously assess the ventilations.

Question 6

How might you best communicate with your patient about assisting with ventilation?

Constant, clear communication with your patient is key in successful ventilation assistance. It is imperative that you remain calm and reassuring during this crisis. Additionally, you should be familiar with the proper techniques for bag-mask ventilation in both one- and two-rescuer situations.

Patient Care Report for Mr. Donnelly

EMS Patient Care Report (PCR)

Date: 12-25-2010	Incident No.: 126551	Nature of Call: Difficulty breathing	Location: 135 Sycamore Street	
Dispatched: 2054	En Route: 2056	At Scene: 2101	Transport: 2116	At Hospital: 2129	In Service: 2154

Patient Information

Age: 77 years
Sex: Male
Weight (in kg [lb]): 81 kg (178 lb)

Allergies: Morphine and latex
Medications: Daily vitamins, furosemide (Lasix), polycarbophil (Fibercon), warfarin (Coumadin), diclofenac (Voltaren ophthalmic), and hydroxyzine (Atarax)
Past Medical History: Triple bypass, CHF, cataract surgery, hypertension, occasional constipation
Chief Complaint: Difficulty breathing

Vital Signs

Time	BP	Pulse	Respirations	SpO₂
2104	162/96	120 regular and weak	36, shallow and labored	88% on home oxygen at 4 L/min
2113	150/88	120 regular and weak	40, shallow and labored	91% with high-flow oxygen

EMS Treatment (circle all that apply)

Oxygen @ **15** L/min via (circle one): NC **(NRM)** **(Bag-mask Device)**	**(Assisted Ventilation)**	Airway Adjunct **(NPA)**	CPR
Defibrillation	Bleeding Control	Bandaging	Splinting	Other:

Narrative

Dispatched to the scene of a 77-year-old man with difficulty breathing. On arrival at the scene we were greeted by the patient's son. A faint odor of urine was present in the home. The patient was found sitting in his bedroom in the tripod position with labored breathing. The patient's son informed us of his father's history of congestive heart failure. Patient was receiving home oxygen, 4 L/min via a nasal cannula. Patient was unable to speak in complete sentences, but was alert and oriented to person, place, day, and event. On initial assessment, the airway was found to be open. Breathing was very labored with accessory muscle use present. Pulses were weak and rapid in both upper extremities. Trauma was ruled out based on the history given by the patient's son. Initial GCS score was 15. Patient was immediately administered high-flow oxygen via a nonrebreathing mask. The patient's son confirmed that the patient does not have a do not resuscitate order. En route to the hospital, an NPA was inserted and ventilations were assisted with a bag-valve mask device. ALS was dispatched, but were delayed by train at railroad crossing, so patient was transported by BLS. EMT Scott met up with us to assist in caring for the patient. Ventilations were assisted during the rest of the transport to the emergency department. GCS was 11 on arrival in the ED. Patient transferred to the hospital staff. **End of report**

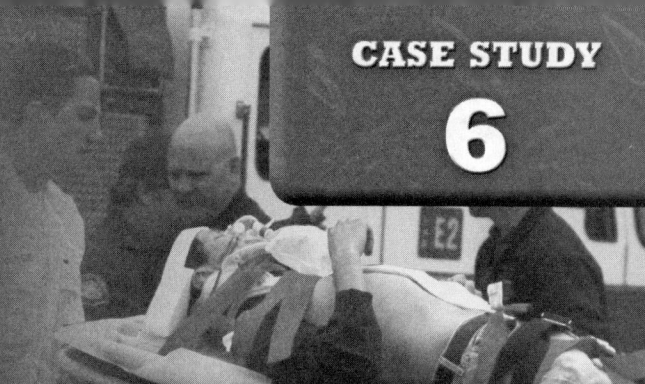

CASE STUDY 6

Shock

Arborist With a Fall Injury

On a brisk autumn day, you and your partner can hear the wind beginning to pick up outside of the fire house. The morning's forecast called for increasing winds and decreasing temperatures. The temperature overnight dropped and it is now 40°F at 0900 hours. The meteorologist on the local news channel is reporting that wind speeds are now up to 20 miles per hour. You cannot help but wonder what is in store for you today with the inclement weather. While you and your partner, Rich, are discussing the weather, the tones sound.

You are dispatched to 777 Westfall Road for a 25-year-old man who fell from a tree during trimming. You recognize the address as the location of a popular park. The bystander who called 9-1-1 reported that the patient fell a great distance to the ground and was responsive but in a lot of pain. Your time out for this call is 0908 hours. En route to the call, you receive an update from the dispatcher. Bystanders now state that the patient has become restless, is reporting increasing pain, and appears pale.

Question 1
Considering the dispatch information, what types of injuries do you anticipate?

Question 2
What specific scene safety considerations should you be concerned about?

You arrive on scene to find the patient lying on the cold, grassy ground in a supine position. It is apparent that your patient has an open airway when he says "hi" to you, and is tracking you as you approach. He reports severe pain to his pelvic area. You introduce yourself to the patient and ask him his name. He tells you his name is George. Rich stabilizes the patient's head as you instruct the patient to lie still. You assess George's level of consciousness and find him to be alert and oriented to person, place, time, and event. Witnesses confirm that George fell approximately 30 feet (11 meters) from the tree to the ground. He landed on his right side.

After hearing this, you perform a primary assessment on George **Table 1**. You place him on high-flow oxygen because of the mechanism of injury (MOI). You expose George's chest, find nothing remarkable, and cover him back up. During your circulation check, you note some minor bleeding to the right leg, but it does not appear to be life threatening. He appears to be very anxious and despite his efforts to remain calm, he tells you the pain in his pelvis is becoming unbearable. He also reports nausea.

Table 1 — Primary Assessment Findings for George

General impression	25-year-old man with fall injury.
Chief complaint	Severe pelvic pain, nausea.
Level of consciousness	Alert and oriented to person, place, time, and event.
Airway	Intact.
Breathing	Equal bilateral chest rise.
Circulation	Skin is pale, slightly moist, and cool.
	Regular, rapid pulses present in both upper extremities.
	No major bleeding noted.
Life threats	Assess for possible head injury.
Pertinent negatives	No broken teeth or other possible airway obstructions.
	No pain with breathing.
Pupils	Dilated 4 mm, equal and reactive to light.
Pain	Pelvic region is 10 on a scale of 1 to 10.
Glasgow coma scale (GCS)	Score: 15 (eye opening, 4; verbal response, 5; motor response, 6).
Interventions	High-flow oxygen via a nonrebreathing mask.

Question 3

On the basis of your primary assessment findings, how would you categorize the priority of this patient and why?

You perform a rapid trauma assessment on this patient **Table 2**. A rescue unit from your company pulls up and the crew members offer their assistance. You ask them to bring you the backboard, a cervical collar, straps, and blankets. Additionally, you ask them to turn the heat on in the patient compartment of the ambulance.

Table 2	Rapid Trauma Assessment Findings for George
Mechanism of injury/nature of illness	Significant fall from a tree.
Level of consciousness	Patient is alert and oriented to person, place, day, and event.
Head/neck/face	Unremarkable for deformities, contusions, abrasions, punctures, penetrations, paradoxical motion in the chest, burns, tenderness, lacerations, or swelling (DCAP-BTLS).
	Patient denies any pain to head/neck/face.
	No blood or fluid coming from ears/eyes/nose/mouth.
	Pupils are dilated 4 mm and are equal and reactive to light.
	Patient was wearing an approved arborist helmet at the time of the fall. The helmet was removed by coworkers and had a visible crack to the front of it.
Chest	Unremarkable for DCAP-BTLS.
	Patient denies any pain to the chest.
	Equal expansion bilaterally with no crepitus.
	Patient denies difficulty breathing.
	Lung sounds are clear and equal bilaterally.
Abdomen	Very tender and distention is noted.
	No rigidity or pulsating masses noted.
	No visible bleeding or discoloration noted.
Pelvis/genitalia	Significant pain on palpation.
	Pain is 10 on a scale of 1 to 10.
	Unstable pelvis with crepitus and swollen abdominal quadrants.
Lower extremities	Pain, tenderness, and swelling to the lower part of the right leg and laceration with minor bleeding.
	Left leg is sore with bruising noted but no bleeding.
Upper extremities	Tenderness to the right upper arm with swelling noted.
	Pain to both hands with bruising seen on the palms.
Back	Tenderness down the spine but no pain or deformities.
Glasgow coma scale (GCS)	Score: 15 (eye opening, 4; verbal response, 5; motor response, 6).

Because of the inclement weather, you decide it would be best to obtain a SAMPLE history, including signs and symptoms, allergies, medications, pertinent past medical history, last oral intake, and events leading up to the illness or injury **Table 3**, and ascertain baseline vital signs **Table 4** once inside the warmth and shelter of the ambulance.

Question 4

How would you stabilize this patient's pelvis before moving him to the backboard?

Table 3 — SAMPLE History for George

Signs and symptoms	Painful, distended abdomen.
	Painful, swollen, right lower leg with minor bleeding from a suturable laceration approximately 10 cm in length.
	Pale, moist skin.
	Tenderness noted in spine.
	Pelvic instability and pain.
Allergies	Codeine
Medications	Varenicline (Chantix)
Pertinent past medical history	History of smoking, prehypertension.
Last oral intake	Breakfast at around 0630, which consisted of caffeinated coffee and an egg, cheese, and sausage bagel sandwich.
Events leading up to the illness or injury	Patient was trimming an oak tree approximately 30 ft (11 m) up when the branch he was using as his anchor point broke. Patient was holding the chain saw in his hands at the time and may have cut his leg on the way down. Patient and coworkers confirm no loss of consciousness.

Table 4 — Baseline Vital Signs for George

Respirations	26 breaths/min and shallow
Pulse	Radial pulse, 135 beats/min and regular
Skin	Cool, moist, and pale
Blood pressure	120/82 mm Hg
Oxygen saturation	97% on high-flow oxygen

George's pelvis was stabilized and he was secured to a backboard for transfer to the awaiting ambulance. While you are assessing the patient's vital signs, your partner switches the portable oxygen to the on-board cylinder. You ask Rich how far away advanced life support (ALS) is and he tells you that their estimated time of arrival is approximately 6 minutes. You ask them to rendezvous with you en route because you think this patient may need pain control and fluid replacement during the 20-minute transport to the nearest trauma facility.

Question 5

What transport considerations should you make for this patient and why?

Once you are en route to the trauma center, you perform a secondary assessment Table 5.

Table 5 — Secondary Assessment Findings for George

Level of consciousness	Patient continues to moan and cry out in pain but level of consciousness has deteriorated.
Airway	Remains intact.
Breathing	Shallow respiration with equal expansion.
Circulation	Skin is pale, moist, and cool.
	Regular, rapid pulse in upper extremities.
Head/neck/face	A small bruise is forming under the patient's jaw line, and a minor abrasion to his left cheek has become apparent.
	Patient still denies any pain to head/neck/face.
	No blood or fluid from the eyes, ears, nose, mouth.
	Pupils are sluggish to react.
Chest	Unremarkable for DCAP-BTLS.
	Patient denies any pain to the chest.
	Patient continues to have equal expansion bilaterally with no crepitus.
	Lung sounds are clear and equal bilaterally.
	Patient denies difficulty breathing.
Abdomen	Upper abdominal quadrants are now tender and there is noticeable distention.
	Lower abdominal quadrants are very tender and distention is noted.
	A large hematoma is now beginning to form in the lower left quadrant. Abdomen is diffusely tender and patient rates pain as 10 out of 10.
Pelvis/genitalia	Significant pain on palpation, pain remains at 10 out of 10.
	Unstable pelvis with crepitus and swollen abdominal quadrants.
	Bleeding from the genitalia and rectum is noted and is apparent by the amount soaked into his pants.
Lower extremities	Tenderness, swelling, and minor bleeding to the right lower extremity.
	Left leg is mildly tender but no bleeding or swelling is noted.
Upper extremities	Tenderness to the right upper arm, which now shows both swelling and bruising.
	Pain to both hands with bruising on the palms.
Back	Tenderness down the spine but no major pain or deformities.
Pain	Pelvic region is 10 on a scale of 1 to 10.
Glasgow coma scale (GCS)	Score: 13 (eye opening, 4; verbal response, 4; motor response, 5).

In addition to the findings in the secondary assessment, you also obtain another set of vital signs (Table 6).

Table 6 Second Set of Vital Signs for George

Respirations	28 breaths/min, rapid and shallow
Pulse	135 beats/min and regular
Skin	Cool, moist, and pale
Blood pressure	110/78 mm Hg
Oxygen saturation	98% on high-flow oxygen

Question 6

On the basis of the findings of the secondary assessment, what other treatment should be given at this time?

You treat the open leg wound to the right leg with a sterile bandage and a padded splint. You have added trauma dressing to the groin area to assist in the controlling of bleeding. You also apply several cold packs to the area to help with bleeding control and minor pain management. At this time the ALS ambulance has arrived.

The arriving paramedic is Shannon. As your driver is assisting Shannon with her equipment in the rig, you brief her on George's condition. Shannon sets up her equipment to obtain intravenous access.

Question 7

What is your role now that ALS has arrived?

After Shannon administers Fentanyl, George calms down and stops complaining of pain. You check his airway, breathing, and circulation again and ask how he is feeling. He now reports his level of pain to be 4 out of 10 and says he is still feeling a bit cold. You cover him with two more wool blankets, turn up the heat in the patient compartment, and reassess his vital signs for a third time (Table 7).

Table 7 Third Set of Vital Signs for George

Respirations	24 breaths/min and regular
Pulse	112 beats/min and regular
Skin	Cool, moist, and pale
Blood pressure	112/80 mm Hg
Oxygen saturation	99% on high-flow oxygen

It seems that the oxygen, morphine, and blankets have helped stabilize the patient's condition during transport to the trauma center. You continue to talk to George to reassess his level of consciousness. As tired as he may be, you would prefer he does not fall asleep. Rich tells you that you are 4 minutes from the emergency department.

Question 8

What could you do while you are treating and transporting George to the trauma center?

You call ahead to Memorial Hospital to let them know that you have a trauma patient with multisystem trauma and a possible pelvic fracture. You give a member of the emergency department staff your patient's last set of vital signs and tell her that you have a paramedic on board.

On arrival, you are escorted quickly to the trauma bay where several nurses and physicians are awaiting your arrival. Shannon gives staff members an update on the patient and you assist in lifting the board to the trauma bed. After waiting to see if the emergency department staff has any further questions for you, you wish George well and leave the trauma bay. Before you leave the hospital, you take the time to remove your gloves properly and wash your hands at one of the sinks. You assist Shannon and Rich in cleaning up the back of the ambulance, putting equipment away, and restocking the items used.

Question 9

What special documentation considerations do you have for this particular call?

Case Analysis

- **Question 1**

    Considering the dispatch information, what types of injuries do you anticipate?

    This call has a high probability for multisystem trauma because of the MOI and the distance of the fall. Responders should be alert to possible head, neck, spine, and thoracic trauma. Depending on how this patient landed and what he hit on the way down, he is a potential candidate for extremity trauma as well. Considering the current weather conditions, he is also a potential candidate for hypothermia and shock.

- **Question 2**

    What specific scene safety considerations should you be concerned about?

    Because of the high wind, you should be concerned about any falling debris from the tree as well as the cold temperatures. Providers also run the risk of hypothermia on calls.

- **Question 3**

    On the basis of your primary assessment findings, how would you categorize the priority of this patient and why?

Although the patient's airway and breathing are intact during the initial assessment, his circulatory status indicates early or compensated shock (cool, moist, pale skin; tachycardia; restlessness; and adequate systolic blood pressure). Compensated shock is the body's first response to hypoperfusion as a result of internal or external hemorrhage. When perfusion is decreased, the heart tries to compensate by increasing the speed at which it pumps. The body further compensates by shunting blood from the skin and extremities to the vital organs, such as the heart, brain, and kidneys. This is why the skin will appear pale or lacking in color and may be cool and moist. The body is also attempting to keep the core warm. In addition, the gastrointestinal tract is another common area from which blood will be shunted away in times of duress. Be prepared for nausea and vomiting. Pupil reaction may be affected by drug overdose, low oxygen levels (hypoxia), or inadequate tissue perfusion (trauma is one possible reason for inadequate tissue perfusion).

■ Question 4

How would you stabilize this patient's pelvis before moving him to the backboard?

Pelvic fractures are cause for great concern because they have the potential for causing life-threatening internal bleeding. Therefore, it is essential to properly manage any pelvic fractures in the field. The goal of pelvic fracture management is to prevent further internal blood loss and support the pelvis by keeping it stabilized and immobile. Patients who suffer a pelvic fracture often have intra-abdominal bleeding. External stabilization is essential to any unstable pelvic fracture in the field, especially those accompanied by hypoperfusion. To manage a pelvic fracture there are several commercial devices available on the market. If your organization does not have a commercial device, then one can be made from cloth sheets or cotton blankets, if local protocol allows. This technique is known as the pelvic wrap technique or pelvic sheet wrap. Like other forms of splinting, the goal behind the pelvic wrap is to stabilize the fractured bone fragments to prevent further injury and blood loss. The pelvic wrap method works by tamponading the blood within the pelvic compartment and stabilizing any unstable bone piece, thus preventing further injury. Whether you use a commercially available device or a sheet wrap, these methods will provide for circumferential compression to stabilize the fracture or fractures of the pelvis.

■ Question 5

What transport considerations should you make for this patient and why?

Because of the severity of this patient's injuries, the MOI, and his vital signs, this patient needs to be transported to a trauma center as soon as possible for more definitive care. Other transport considerations should include keeping the patient warm, supplying high-flow oxygen, minimizing bleeding, and providing a smooth ride to the hospital.

■ Question 6

On the basis of the findings of the secondary assessment, what other treatment should be given at this time?

Control bleeding with sterile dressings to the leg and splint for immobilization. Trauma dressings should be used to control bleeding to the groin, and the pelvic girdle should be immobilized.

■ Question 7

What is your role now that ALS has arrived?

Your role as a basic life support (BLS) provider should continue with ALS personnel. Oftentimes, EMTs may feel that their role as caregiver takes a backseat when paramedics or other ALS providers are present. This could not be further from the truth. BLS and ALS personnel should work together as a team to manage patient care priorities. You can continue to assess the patient alongside ALS. This may include continuing a patient assessment, history taking, reassessment, proper communication with the patient, and supplying the ALS provider with information regarding any changes to the patient's condition. Some basic providers will assist with ALS skills, such as setting up an intravenous bag for fluid replacement.

■ Question 8

What could you do while you are treating and transporting George to the trauma center?

Communicating with your patient is a priority in continuing care. In addition, reassessing mental status and vital signs, and calling ahead to the trauma center are all responsibilities that fall under the EMT's scope of practice and can be done for the remainder of the transport.

■ Question 9

What special documentation considerations do you have for this particular call?

Whereas all calls require thorough documentation, some calls, such as this one, may require more in-depth documentation. For example, a detailed scene description would be valuable for the continuation of care at the hospital. Because it is not possible or realistic for the hospital staff to visually see the scene, your words in writing will provide an image and backdrop for the call. Another aspect of documentation that is important for this patient would be the alterations in level of consciousness, all vital sign changes, and responses to treatment.

44 Shock

Patient Care Report for George

EMS Patient Care Report (PCR)

Date: 10-03-2011	Incident No.: 123561	Nature of Call: Fall from tree		Location: 777 Westfall Road	
Dispatched: 0906	En Route: 0908	At Scene: 0914	Transport: 0926	At Hospital: 0949	In Service: 1000

Patient Information

Age: 25 years
Sex: Male
Weight (in kg [lb]): 75 kg (165 lb)

Allergies: codeine
Medications: varenicline (Chantix)
Past Medical History: History of smoking, prehypertension
Chief Complaint: Pelvic pain and nausea

Vital Signs

Time: 0925	BP: 120/82	Pulse: 135 and regular	Respirations: 26 and shallow	SpO_2: 97% on high-flow oxygen
Time: 0931	BP: 110/78	Pulse: 135 and regular	Respirations: 28 rapid and shallow	SpO_2: 98% on high-flow oxygen
Time: 0937	BP: 112/80	Pulse: 112 and regular	Respirations: 24 and regular	SpO_2: 99% on high-flow oxygen

EMS Treatment
(circle all that apply)

Oxygen @ **15** L/min via (circle one): NC **(NRM)** Bag-Valve Device

Assisted Ventilation | Airway Adjunct | CPR

Defibrillation | **(Bleeding Control)** | **(Bandaging)** | **(Splinting)** R Leg and Pelvis | **(Other:)** Cold Therapy

Narrative

Dispatched to the scene of a 25-year-old man who fell about 30 feet (11 meters) out of a tree to a grassy surface. On arrival, patient found lying supine on the ground. Patient presented with a patent airway. Patient complained of severe pain to the pelvis. Manual cervical spine stabilization initiated immediately by Rich. Patient was found to be alert and oriented to person, place, time, and event. Bystander confirmed that the patient fell approximately 30 feet, landed on his right side, and did not lose consciousness. Airway was intact and no broken teeth or obstructions noted in the mouth. Patient's breathing was equal bilaterally and he denied any pain with respiration. Patient was placed on high-flow oxygen via nonrebreathing mask. Assessment of the chest reveals no DCAP-BTLS. Minor bleeding was noted to the right lower extremity. Skin was noted as pale, moist, and cool to the touch. Patient appeared anxious and complained of increased pain to the pelvis and nausea. Rapid assessment performed prior to moving patient onto backboard. Rapid trauma assessment revealed abdominal tenderness and distention. Pain in the pelvis was rated as 10/10 and was accompanied by instability and crepitus. Swelling was noted to the lower part of the right leg with minor bleeding. Left leg was sore but no bleeding or swelling was noted. Tenderness noted to the right upper extremity and pain to both hands with bruising to the palms. Tenderness noted down the back but no major deformities. GCS score was 15 at that time. Pelvis was stabilized with a pelvic wrap using cravats and towels. Patient was placed on a backboard to be moved to gurney in warm ambulance. Patient stated he was trimming an oak tree when the branch he was using as his anchor point broke. Patient was holding a chainsaw in his hands at the time of the fall. A secondary assessment was performed in the ambulance. Small bruises were visible to the face along with abrasions. Patient still denied any pain to the head, neck, or face. Chest was still unremarkable and patient denied any pain or difficulty breathing. All four abdominal quadrants were noted as tender and distended and a large hematoma began to form over the lower abdominal quadrants. Pain to the abdominal area increased. Pain to the pelvis remained at 10 out of 10. Exposure of the pelvic region revealed significant bleeding from the genitalia and rectum. Trauma dressings applied to this region and pelvic splint was readjusted. Pain was still present in the lower right leg with minor bleeding, which was controlled with a dressing and gauze. A padded splint was used to stabilize the right leg. Cold packs were applied to the right leg to help control bleeding and swelling. Left leg noted as sore but no DCAP-BTLS noted. There continued to be tenderness to the right upper arm and pain and bruising to both palms. Patient's GCS score decreased to 13. Level of consciousness was noted as decreasing with moaning and crying out in pain. ALS Unit 26, Shannon, met up with crew for transport to hospital. After pain relief administered by Medic 26, patient reported being in less pain and reported his pain as 4 out of 10. Vital signs reassessed after pain medication administered by paramedic. Patient reported feeling cold so more blankets were added for warmth. Lehigh Valley Emergency Department was notified of impending arrival of patient and crew. Patient and crew moved immediately to bed 1 in the trauma bay. Crew transferred care of patient to the emergency department staff. **End of report**

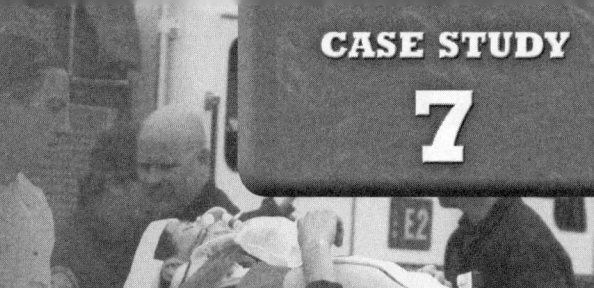

CASE STUDY 7

Respiratory Emergencies

Girl With Asthma

With today's high humidity and heavy pollen count, your allergies are making it difficult to focus and stay alert. You are hoping that the air conditioning in the ambulance does not stop working. The tones sound and you and your partner, Tyrese, are dispatched to a call at 2245 Driving Park Avenue, Apartment 2B, for a 9-year-old girl with difficulty breathing. You are advised that advanced life support (ALS) is also en route. Dispatch also advises that the child has a history of asthma. Time out is 1302.

Question 1

What type of medication(s) are most often prescribed for persons with asthma?

On arrival you are greeted by a woman who appears to be in her early 50s. She is waving her arms frantically in the driveway. You grab your equipment and follow her up the back staircase. On the way up the stairs she tells you that her name is Henrietta and that her granddaughter is having a bad attack. Henrietta is very concerned and she explains that her 9-year-old granddaughter has a history of asthma and is working hard to breathe. She says, "Hurry, please hurry!"

Question 2

Does knowing that the patient is only 9 years old and not an adult change your treatment plan for this call? Why or why not?

You ask Tyrese to check the status of ALS backup. He tells you that ALS is about 10 minutes out.

By the time you enter the upstairs apartment, you are drenched in sweat. The air inside the apartment feels very hot, heavy, and still. Henrietta takes you to the bathroom where you find the 9-year-old girl sitting in the tripod position on the toilet lid. You see obvious nasal flaring and intercostal retractions. A baby is sitting in an infant carrier on the floor of the bathroom.

Question 3

What is your immediate treatment plan for this child?

Respiratory Emergencies

The grandmother tells you that the patient's name is Tasha and that she has had increasing trouble breathing for about an hour. She was hoping Tasha's mother would be home from work by now so she could take her to the doctor without having to take the baby. You introduce yourself to Tasha. She replies, "Hi. It's ... hard ... to ... breathe." You can see that she is very tired. She is speaking in two- to three-word sentences and has a look of fear in her eyes.

Question 4

What signs and symptoms might you expect to see in this patient?

As you begin to gather a SAMPLE history from the grandmother, including signs and symptoms, allergies, medications, pertinent past medical history, last oral intake, and events leading up to the illness or injury, you assess that her oxygen saturation is only 89% on room air Table 1 . Based on the nature of the call and Tasha's signs and symptoms, you administer high-flow oxygen to Tasha. Tyrese comes back upstairs with the pediatric bag and a stair chair.

Table 1 SAMPLE History for Tasha

Signs and symptoms	Difficulty breathing.
	Retractions and nasal flaring.
	Perioral (around the mouth) cyanosis.
Allergies	No known drug allergies.
Medications	Albuterol (Proventil) inhaler and nebulized albuterol.
Pertinent past medical history	Asthma, premature birth at 30 weeks of gestation.
Last oral intake	Breakfast around 0900 hours consisting of milk, cereal, and a banana.
Events leading up to the illness or injury	Walking up the flight of stairs to their apartment in the heat and humidity about 2 hours prior to 9-1-1 dispatch.

Question 5

Which questions about the patient's condition would be important to ask before you begin any further treatment?

You perform an assessment on Tasha and gather some important medical information from Tasha's grandmother Table 2 and obtain a set of baseline vital signs Table 3 .

Table 2 — Primary Assessment Findings for Tasha

General impression	9-year-old girl experiencing difficulty breathing.
Chief complaint	Difficulty breathing.
Level of consciousness	Alert to surroundings.
	Responds in two-to-three word sentences but appears oriented.
Airway	Patent at the moment.
Breathing	High-flow oxygen administered.
	Chest expansion is equal but shallow and labored.
	Visible retractions noted at the clavicles and along the rib cage.
	Nasal flaring.
	Audible wheezes.
	Expiratory wheezes in all fields.
Circulation	Strong, rapid pulses present in both upper extremities.
	No external bleeding.
Life threats	Difficulty breathing due to an asthma attack.
Interventions	Oxygen administered.
	After obtaining a medical history, medication administered.
	Further assessment, treatment, and transport needed.
Pain	Cannot articulate at the moment.
Pulse oximetry	Initially 89% on room air, now 95% on high-flow oxygen.
Glasgow coma scale (GCS)	Score: 15 (eye opening, 4; verbal response, 5; motor response, 6).
Recent immunizations	Measles, mumps, rubella, and varicella.
Mechanism of injury/nature of illness	Asthma attack.
Pertinent negatives	No trauma either today or recently.
How often does she experience asthma attacks?	A few times a year.
When was her last asthma attack?	About 3 months ago while at school.
Has she ever been hospitalized for an asthma attack?	No.
Any recent illness?	No.
Has she ever needed to go to the emergency department for an asthma attack?	Yes.
Has she ever needed to be intubated before for an asthma attack?	Grandmother didn't know.
How long has she been wheezing?	Grandmother didn't know.
Any corticosteroid use in the past 24 hours?	No.

Respiratory Emergencies

Question 6

What are the six rights of medication administration?

Tasha had a dose of her metered-dose inhaler (MDI) about 1 hour ago and her grandmother tells you that the MDI is now empty. Tasha has an at-home nebulizer but she does not have it at her grandmother's house today. You opt to give her a small-volume nebulizer (SVN) treatment, which you have in the pediatric bag. You are carrying a pediatric mask in your gear, so you are able to administer the SVN while transferring the patient to the ambulance. With Tasha's severe work of breathing, you decide it is in her best interest to move quickly to the ambulance for further reevaluation and treatment.

After putting Tasha on the stair chair and securing her with the straps, you ask her grandmother if she has a favorite stuffed animal or toy that would be appropriate to bring. Tasha's grandmother grabs her teddy bear and hands it to her. Henrietta tells you she will have to get a ride to the hospital later because Tasha's mother has her car. She would like you to take Tasha to Miami Children's Hospital.

Paramedic Darrin meets you outside. He is all set up with his equipment and asks you for a history on the patient. Now that Tasha has completed her SVN treatment, you begin to reassess her **Table 4**.

After reaching the cool interior of the ambulance and administering high-concentration oxygen and the SVN treatment, you are satisfied with the improvement in the patient's condition. About 5 minutes away from Miami Children's Hospital, Tasha even smiles and you breathe a sigh of relief.

Table 3 Baseline Vital Signs for Tasha

Respirations	36 breaths/min and shallow
	Increased work of breathing
	Nasal flaring and retractions
	Audible wheezing
Pulse	122 beats/min and regular
Skin	Warm and moist
Blood pressure	98/68 mm Hg
Oxygen saturation	95% on high-flow oxygen

Table 4 Secondary Assessment Findings for Tasha

Level of consciousness	Alert and oriented to person, place, time, and event.
Airway	Patent.
Breathing	High-flow oxygen administered.
	Nebulized bronchodilator administered.
	Chest expansion is equal and unlabored.
	Retractions and nasal flaring have diminished significantly.
	No audible sounds.
	Auscultation reveals improvement to expiratory wheezes.
Circulation	Strong, rapid pulses present in both upper extremities.
	No external bleeding noted.
Life threats	Breathing difficulties due to an asthma attack have diminished after oxygen and SVN treatment.
Capillary refill	Less than 2 seconds.
Pain	No pain.
Glasgow coma scale (GCS)	Score: 15 (eye opening, 4; verbal response, 5; motor response, 6).

Case Analysis

Question 1

What type of medication(s) are most often prescribed for persons with asthma?

People with known asthma are most often prescribed inhalers, which are designed to alleviate difficulty breathing associated with an asthma attack. These inhaler medications are also known as bronchodilators because they dilate (open up) the tiny airway passages in the base of the lungs. Bronchodilator medications frequently come in the form of MDIs. MDIs are small, handheld devices that hold the medication and can be aerosolized when dispensed Figure 1. The metered-dose inhaler provides a set amount of medication each time it is depressed. This way the patient gets the same amount each time and does not need to measure the medication during a time of need or crisis Table 5.

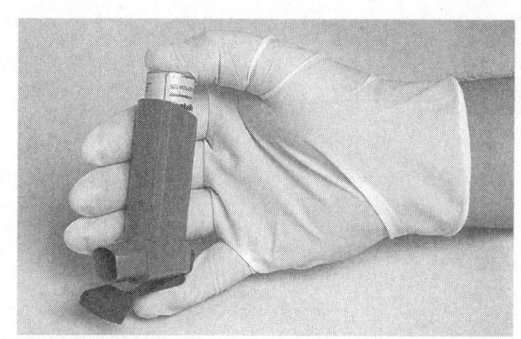

Figure 1 Metered-dose inhalers are miniature spray canisters used to direct medications through the mouth and into the lungs.

Table 5 Respiratory Inhalation Medications

Medication			Indications			Use: Acute Versus Chronic Disease	
Generic Drug Name	Trade Names	Action	Asthma	Bronchitis	COPD	Acute	Chronic
Albuterol	Proventil, Ventolin, Volmax	Dilates bronchioles	Yes	Yes	Yes	Yes	No
Beclomethasone dipropionate	Beclovent, Beconase, Qvar, Vanceril	Anti-inflammatory, reduces swelling	Yes	No	No	No	Yes
Cromolyn sodium	Crolom, Gastrocom, Intal, Nasalcrom	Decreases release of histamines	Yes	No	No	No	Yes
Fluticasone propionate	Cutivate, Flonase, Flovent	Anti-inflammatory, reduces swelling	Yes	No	No	No	Yes
Fluticasone propionate, salmeterol xinafoate	Advair Diskus	Decreases secretions	Yes	No	No	No	Yes
Ipratropium bromide	Atrovent	Dilates bronchioles	Yes	Yes	Yes	Yes	No
Metaproterenol sulfate	Alupent, Metaprel	Dilates bronchioles	Yes	Yes	Yes	Yes	No
Salmeterol xinafoate	Serevent	Dilates bronchioles	Yes	Yes	Yes	No	Yes

Question 2

Does knowing that the patient is only 9 years old and not an adult change your treatment plan for this call? Why or why not?

EMS and first responders do not usually have as much hands-on experience working with children in emergencies, so the providers may not be as comfortable as they would be when treating adult patients. With that said, there are some specific pediatric considerations to take into account for this call. To begin, this 9-year-old child may require pediatric-sized airway management equipment. In addition, you should be prepared to immediately dispatch an ALS provider in case the child goes into complete respiratory failure. The pediatric airway presents with many anatomic differences (large tongue, small glottis) that make maintaining it, especially in time of crisis, a particularly difficult challenge. All equipment, including the blood pressure cuff, needs to be appropriately sized to give more accurate diagnostics. Finally, the pediatric patient assessment requires special skills and training. Many sources suggest that it would be prudent to use the pediatric assessment triangle to assist with your general approach and assessment.

Question 3

What is your immediate treatment plan for this child?

Immediate treatment for this child should focus on airway management. Ensuring and maintaining a patent airway is the number one priority in treating a patient with asthma. Immediately administer high-flow oxygen while finishing your assessment and obtaining a complete patient history.

Question 4

What signs and symptoms might you expect to see in this patient?

Patients with asthma may present with the following:
- Appearance of anxiety, fear, or even panic
- Shortness of breath/difficulty breathing and/or air hunger (where the patient appears starved for air)
- Changes in level of consciousness because of lack of oxygen to the brain
- Nasal flaring
- Intercostal, clavicular, or substernal retractions
- Tripod positioning
- Audible wheezing or wheezing on auscultation (usually during the expiratory phase of breathing)
- Cyanosis to the lips and/or nail beds
- Head bobbing
- Mottled skin

Question 5

Which questions about the patient's condition would be important to ask before you begin any further treatment?

- Did she suffer any trauma today?
- How long ago was Tasha diagnosed with asthma?
- How long has she had difficulty breathing today?
- Did you do anything to help treat her asthma before calling 9-1-1?
- Is Tasha on any medications? If so, which ones?
- Has she been prescribed any bronchodilators? If so, MDI or nebulized albuterol?
- Has Tasha taken any of her bronchodilators today? If so, how long ago? How much?
- Did those medications work? What were the effects?
- Does Tasha have any allergies to medications?
- What was Tasha doing when her signs and symptoms began?
- How often does she experience asthma attacks?
- When was her last asthma attack?
- Has she ever been hospitalized for an asthma attack?
- Has she ever needed to go to the emergency department for an asthma attack?
- Has she ever needed to be intubated for an asthma attack?
- What does a normal asthma attack look like for Tasha?
- Is she up to date on her immunizations?
- When was the last time she ate/drank anything?

Asking about the patient's specific asthma history gives you an indication for the potential severity of her current asthma attack. It can also give you an idea of how this patient's condition may progress while in your care.

Question 6

What are the six rights of medication administration?

The six rights of medication administration are:
- Right patient
- Right medication
- Right route
- Right dose
- Right time
- Right documentation

This check before administering medications is crucial to the safe administration of medications to any patient, whether he or she is in the hospital or in the prehospital setting. Medication errors can be eliminated with proper checks and rechecks.

Patient Care Report for Tasha

EMS Patient Care Report (PCR)

Date: 07-16-2011	Incident No.: 126322	Nature of Call: Difficulty breathing	Location: 2245 Driving Park Avenue, Apartment 2B	
Dispatched: 1300	En Route: 1302	At Scene: 1324	Transport: 1324	At Hospital: 1337	In Service: 1409

Patient Information

Age: 9 years
Sex: Female
Weight (in kg [lb]): 37 kg (82 lb)

Allergies: No known drug allergies
Medications: Albuterol (Proventil) inhaler and nebulized albuterol
Past Medical History: Asthma, premature birth at 30 weeks
Chief Complaint: Difficulty breathing

Vital Signs

Time: 1314	BP: 98/68	Pulse: 122 and regular	Respirations: 36, shallow and labored with nasal flaring and retractions	SpO$_2$: 95% on O$_2$
Time:	BP:	Pulse:	Respirations:	SpO$_2$:
Time:	BP:	Pulse:	Respirations:	SpO$_2$:

EMS Treatment
(circle all that apply)

Oxygen @ <u>15</u> L/min via (circle one): NC (NRM) Bag-Mask Device	Assisted Ventilation	Airway Adjunct	CPR
Defibrillation	Bleeding Control	Bandaging	Splinting	(Other:) SVN

Narrative

Dispatched to a multifamily dwelling for a report of a girl having an asthma attack. On our arrival to the second floor apartment, patient's grandmother escorted us in to the bathroom, where the 9-year-old girl was seated on the toilet lid, in a tripod position, exhibiting signs of difficulty breathing. Nasal flaring and retractions were present as was cyanosis around the lips. There was no air conditioning inside the apartment. Patient was alert but was speaking in two- to three-word sentences. Airway was patent. High-flow oxygen immediately administered via NRM. Chest expansion was shallow, labored, and equal bilaterally. Retractions were noted around the clavicles. Audible wheezes were heard without the use of a stethoscope. Strong, rapid pulses were present in both upper extremities. SVN treatment was administered after ascertaining that the patient is not allergic to the medication. Patient was moved to the ambulance via a stair chair. Patient's grandmother said she'd meet us at Miami Children's Hospital. Paramedic Darrin met us in the ambulance. A secondary assessment was performed in the ambulance. Retractions and nasal flaring had diminished. Audible wheezing had also diminished. Pulses remained strong and rapid in both upper extremities. No external bleeding was noted. Capillary refill was 2 seconds. Patient denied any pain. Oxygen saturation was 97% on oxygen and after the SVN treatment. Patient became more talkative en route to Miami Children's Hospital. Patient remained alert and oriented throughout transport. Patient left in the care of hospital staff. **End of report**

Cardiovascular Emergencies

CASE STUDY 8

Woman With Hot Flashes and Nausea

You and your crew have just finished a nice, quiet lunch at the Highland Park Diner when a call comes in over your radio for a 52-year-old woman in a parking lot with an unknown illness. As you listen to the dispatch you are surprised to find that the address is the same as the diner where you are eating. After a quick scan of the parking lot, you notice a middle-aged woman waving you over to a small sedan. Jorge, your driver, retrieves the ambulance and pulls it up near the patient's car. You and your trainee, Zhack, retrieve your equipment off the ambulance and approach the car. You see a woman in her early- to mid-50s sitting in the front seat of the car. Her friend, Sharissa, is standing next to the open door and begins to tell you what is going on. Sharissa explains that while eating lunch, the woman began to report hot flashes and nausea. Unable to finish her meal, she had excused herself and stated that she was going home to lie down. Sharissa had exited the diner approximately 15 minutes later to find the woman sitting in the front seat of her car, acting confused.

After you introduce yourself, the woman tells you that her name is Taylor. She thinks her friend has made a big deal out of nothing and denies needing the ambulance. You ask her if it is okay to assess her to make sure everything is all right. She seems embarrassed but agrees to a primary assessment **Table 1**. You also use this opportunity to obtain a set of baseline vital signs **Table 2**.

Cardiovascular Emergencies

Table 1 Primary Assessment Findings for Taylor

General impression	52-year-old woman reporting nausea, dizziness, and recurrent hot flashes, general illness.
Chief complaint	Nausea, dizziness, and recurrent hot flashes, general illness.
Mechanism of injury/nature of illness	No trauma. Rule out food poisoning and/or cardiac-related event.
Level of consciousness	Alert and oriented to person, place, day, time, and event.
Airway	Open and patent, free of obvious obstructions.
Breathing	Respirations are within normal limits, chest expansion is equal bilaterally, no chest trauma or evidence of previous chest/cardiac surgery.
Circulation	Strong and slightly irregular radial pulses. Skin is flushed, moist, and warm.
Life threats	Rule out general illness and possible cardiac event.
Pupils	Pupils are equal, round, regular in size, and react properly to light (PEARRL).
Pain	Back pain is a 7 on a scale of 1 to 10.
Glasgow coma scale (GCS)	Score: 15 (eye opening, 4; verbal response, 5; motor response, 6).
Pertinent negatives	Patient denies chest pain or pressure. Patient denies vomiting or losing consciousness. Patient denies trauma.
Interventions	Apply oxygen for dizziness and nausea. Encourage treatment/transport to hospital. Monitor vital signs.

Table 2 Baseline Vital Signs for Taylor

Respirations	22 breaths/min and shallow
Pulse	108 beats/min and irregular
Blood pressure	162/96 mm
Skin	Flushed, moist, and warm
Oxygen saturation	95% on ambient air

You obtain a SAMPLE history, including signs and symptoms, allergies, medications, pertinent past medical history, last oral intake, and events leading up to the illness or injury **Table 3**.

Table 3	SAMPLE History for Taylor
Signs and symptoms	Diaphoretic, flushed skin. Patient reports nausea, hot flashes, dizziness, and general feeling of illness.
Allergies	Codeine.
Medications	Alendronate sodium (Fosamax), atorvastatin (Lipitor), multivitamin, vitamin E.
Pertinent past medical history	High cholesterol, prehypertension, menopausal.
Last oral intake	Lunch about 15 minutes ago.
Events leading up to the illness or injury	Eating lunch with her friend when she had a hot flash and then became nauseated and felt ill.

Question 1

Do you think this patient needs to be transported via ambulance to the hospital? Why or why not?

Taylor keeps saying "This is really being blown out of proportion. I just need to go home and lie down for a bit." You and Jorge are not convinced, and neither is Sharissa. You tell Taylor that you really think she should be checked out at the hospital.

Question 2

What are some ways you might be able to convince patients to go to the hospital if they do not want to go?

After some persuasion from you and Sharissa, Taylor agrees to be transported to the hospital for further evaluation.

Question 3

What type of questions might you ask to obtain a more detailed medical history from the patient?

With Taylor on the gurney in the back of the ambulance, you reassess her condition and ask her more questions about her medical history and current symptoms. After some digging, Taylor admits to not feeling well for about the past 3 to 4 days. She says she just has not felt like herself and has not had much energy. She thought she was just ill with a virus and thought nothing else of it. She explains that today she has had some unusual upper back pain, like a dull ache. En route to the hospital you learn that Taylor thinks she may have passed out after she sat down in her car. She did not want to tell you in front of her friend because she did not want to worry her.

Question 4

With this new assessment information, what would your course of action be for this patient now?

On the basis of the information Taylor has just shared with you, you are concerned that this event could be cardiac related. You communicate to Taylor your thoughts on her possible condition and explain that the course of action will be to rule out any possible cardiac events.

Question 5

Which medication or medications should you administer to this patient and why?

Question 6

Before you administer any medications to a patient, what questions do you need to ask?

You ask Taylor if she has any allergies to medications, specifically aspirin, and also rule out any recent gastrointestinal bleeding, active bleeding, or major surgery. You administer four tablets of baby aspirin and instruct Taylor to chew and swallow them.

Fortunately, Highland Hospital is only about 2 miles from the Highland Park Diner. You have Zhack call ahead to let them know you are on your way in with a patient who may be experiencing a cardiac event. Because of your proximity to the hospital, you do not call for advanced life support (ALS) to meet you.

En route to the emergency department, you perform a secondary assessment on Taylor **Table 4** and obtain a second set of vital signs **Table 5**.

Table 4 — Secondary Assessment Findings for Taylor

Level of consciousness	Remains alert and oriented to person, place, day, time, and event.
Airway	Open and patent.
Breathing	Respirations are within normal limits, chest expansion is equal bilaterally, no chest trauma or evidence of previous chest/cardiac surgery.
	Patient denies any chest pain or pressure.
	Lung sounds are clear.
Circulation	Strong and slightly irregular radial pulses.
	Carotid pulse is strong.
	Dorsalis pedis pulses are present in both lower extremities.
Pupils	Pupils are equal, round, regular in size, and react properly to light (PEARRL).
Pain	Back pain is a 4 on a scale of 1 to 10.
Glasgow coma scale (GCS)	Score: 15 (eye opening, 4; verbal response, 5; motor response, 6).
Life threats	Rule out general illness and possible cardiac event.
Interventions	Continue with oxygen for dizziness and nausea.
	Aspirin administered without any side effects.

Table 5 Second Set of Vital Signs for Taylor

Respirations	16 breaths/min and regular, unlabored
Pulse	98 beats/min and irregular
Blood pressure	150/82 mm Hg
Skin	Flushed, moist, and warm
Oxygen saturation	99% on high-flow oxygen

Taylor remains talkative and is alert and oriented to person, place, time, and event for the brief transport to Highland Hospital. Fortunately, a triage nurse is available within minutes of your arrival and you transfer Taylor to cardiac bed 3R. As you are giving a report to the emergency department doctor, the nurses tell Jorge that the electrocardiogram (ECG) they administered shows she is having an acute myocardial infarction (AMI). Taylor is surprised by this. She thanks you for bringing her in and you say, "Goodbye."

Question 7

In which patient population would you *most* likely suspect *atypical* signs and symptoms of an AMI?

Question 8

Explain what type of outcome your patient might have had if she had not been assessed, treated, and transported to the emergency department.

Case Analysis

■ Question 1

Do you think this patient needs to be transported via ambulance to the hospital? Why or why not?

On the basis of your patient's signs and symptoms as well as her very high blood pressure, this patient should be treated and transported. Her complaint of dizziness means she certainly should not drive herself to the hospital or anywhere else. Considering that signs and symptoms of a heart attack in women often present atypically, it is important for this patient's health for her to be evaluated immediately Table 6 .

Cardiovascular Emergencies

Table 6 Comparison of Typical and Atypical Signs and Symptoms of an Acute Myocardial Infarction (AMI)

Typical Signs and Symptoms of an AMI	Atypical Signs and Symptoms of an AMI
Chest pain or chest pressure in the center of the chest, often described as a squeezing or tightness. Some patients say it feels like something heavy is sitting on their chest.	Syncope (fainting)
	Indigestion
Pain or discomfort in other areas of the upper body, which could include one or both arms, the jaw, back, or stomach.	Altered mental status
	Confusion
Radiating pain to the back.	Fatigue
Diaphoresis (profuse sweating).	Generalized feeling of illness
Shortness of breath or difficulty breathing.	Nausea and/or vomiting
Epigastric pain/indigestion.	Weakness

■ Question 2

What are some ways you might be able to convince patients to go to the hospital if they do not want to go?

When you are caring for patients who are reluctant to be transported to the hospital, it is crucial to convey to them that you are concerned about them. Part of expressing your concern would include informing them why you are concerned. In this case, you are concerned about the patient's dangerously high blood pressure combined with her dizziness. You could let her know that this might be cardiac or stroke related and that her condition could worsen if she does not seek medical help immediately. Because her friend is with her, you could also have her friend try to convince her to seek help.

■ Question 3

What type of questions might you ask to obtain a more detailed medical history from the patient?

Proper treatment of patients involves a thorough assessment, both a physical assessment and a complete medical history assessment. The following questions can be useful:
- Have you been feeling ill lately? If so, for how long?
- Have you changed medications or added any new medications recently?
- Are you compliant with your current medications (meaning do you take them as prescribed)?
- Have you ever felt like this before?

- Have you been to your physician recently for any problems or a routine physical?
- Have you been hospitalized in the past 12 months for any reason?
- Have you experienced any unusual muscle pains lately?
- Is there any increased stress in your life right now?
- How long have you been diagnosed with prehypertension?
- Besides hypertensive medications, have you done anything else to lower your blood pressure?

■ Question 4

With this new assessment information, what would your course of action be for this patient now?

Continue with oxygen administration, assess oxygen saturation, consider calling for ALS depending on transport time to nearest hospital, administer aspirin as appropriate, provide timely transport, monitor vital signs, and reassess the patient.

■ Question 5

Which medication or medications should you administer to this patient and why?

If your patient was prescribed nitroglycerin and had it with her, you could assist in the administration of this medication, per local protocols. If your agency carries aspirin, you may administer it to the patient. Remember that oxygen is also considered a medication. Nitroglycerin is a vasodilator, which would help dilate the coronary arteries, thus making it easier for blood to flow through the coronary arteries to the ischemic heart area. Aspirin has an antiplatelet effect in the blood, thus preventing clots from forming in the arteries. It does not thin the blood as many believe but simply prevents further platelet aggregation.

■ Question 6

Before you administer any medications to a patient, what questions do you need to ask?

- What medications are you currently taking?
- Are you allergic to any medications (specifically to the medication you are going to administer)?
- If you are allergic to the medication, what type of reaction does it cause?
- Have you taken any medications today?
- If so, when? How much? Are they physician prescribed?
- Are you allergic to aspirin?

Aspirin-specific questions:

- Have you had any recent surgery?
- Have you had recent gastrointestinal bleeding or other major bleeding?

■ Question 7

In which patient population would you *most* likely suspect *atypical* signs and symptoms of an AMI?

Atypical signs and symptoms of an AMI occur most frequently in women, persons with diabetes, and geriatric patients.

■ Question 8

Explain what type of outcome your patient might have had if she had not been assessed, treated, and transported to the emergency department.

Had the patient's friend not called 9-1-1, or had the patient chosen not to go to the hospital, her outcome could have been less favorable. One outcome could have been her passing out while driving and crashing her vehicle. Her situation would then have included trauma in addition to her cardiac problem. Had she made it home safely, she could have lost consciousness at home, where she might have been alone with no one to call for help. If someone did find her, she could have been in full cardiac arrest and anoxic (no oxygen). Most importantly, time is a key factor in saving cardiac muscle for a patient who presents with a myocardial infarction. The longer the heart is without oxygen, the higher the chances of irreversible cardiac cell death.

Patient Care Report for Taylor

EMS Patient Care Report (PCR)

Date: 06-12-2010	**Incident No.:** 126551	**Nature of Call:** Illness		**Location:** Highland Park Diner parking lot
Dispatched: 1301	**En Route:** 1301	**At Scene:** 1301	**Transport:** 1315	**At Hospital:** 1320	**In Service:** 1340

Patient Information

Age: 52 years
Sex: Female
Weight (in kg [lb]): 75 kg (172 lb)

Allergies: Codeine
Medications: Alendronate sodium (Fosamax), atorvastatin (Lipitor), multivitamin, vitamin E
Past Medical History: High cholesterol, prehypertension, and menopausal
Chief Complaint: Nausea and dizziness

Vital Signs

Time	BP	Pulse	Respirations	SpO$_2$
1306	162/96	108 and irregular	22 and shallow	95% on room air
1316	150/82	98 and irregular	16 and regular, unlabored	99% on O$_2$

EMS Treatment (circle all that apply)

Oxygen @ <u>15</u> L/min via (circle one): NC **(NRM)** Bag-mask device	Assisted Ventilation	Airway Adjunct	CPR
Defibrillation	Bleeding Control	Bandaging	Splinting	**(Other:)** 4 tablets baby aspirin

Narrative

Dispatched to a call for a 52-year-old woman with an illness in the parking lot of the Highland Park Diner. On arrival, patient found sitting in her car with a friend standing by her side. Patient was complaining of nausea, dizziness, illness, and hot flashes. Patient conscious and alert. Her airway was patent and her breathing was adequate. No evidence of any trauma to the patient. Skin diaphoretic, flushed, and warm. Pulse was strong, rapid, and irregular. Oxygen administered 100% via nonrebreathing mask. Patient stated that she has high cholesterol, prehypertension, and is going through menopause. Patient currently taking alendronate sodium (Fosamax), atorvastatin (Lipitor), multivitamins, and vitamin E. Patient denied any previous cardiac history. Patient last ate approximately 15 minutes prior to our arrival. Patient stated she was eating lunch with her friend when she became ill, believing she was suffering from hot flashes and possible food poisoning. Patient denied any chest pain or chest pressure, denied vomiting and losing consciousness. Patient initially refused transport. Once crew explained their concerns to her, she agreed to go for further evaluation. Patient moved to the ambulance via the gurney. En route to Highland Hospital, patient stated she had not felt well for a few days and had lacked energy. She explained that today was different in that she had some upper back pain, describing it as a dull ache, for approximately 24 hours. At that time, patient admitted that she may have passed out when she got in her car in the parking lot. Four tablets of baby aspirin administered to patient after ruling out an allergy to aspirin and any recent surgery or active bleeding. Back discomfort initially rated as a 7/10. After aspirin administration, pain level fell to a 4/10. Breathing remained unlabored and equal bilaterally. Patient remained calm and talkative en route to Highland Hospital and maintained a GCS score of 15 (4/5/6). On arrival at Highland Hospital, patient was triaged to hospital staff. **End of report**

CASE STUDY 9

Neurologic Emergencies

Woman With a Possible Stroke

The waitress at your favorite diner just brought your dinner out when the call comes in for a 65-year-old woman with a possible stroke. Time out is 1820. On your way to the call, you talk to your trainee, Sharon, who is halfway through an EMT class. Sharon has only been on a few calls and this will be her first call for a possible stroke. You brief her on what to expect.

Question 1

What information would you go over with your trainee en route to this call? What can you tell her to expect for this type of patient?

You enter the single-family residence through the front door and find yourself in the family room. Your patient, Mrs. Messing, is lying on the couch, with her friend, Todd, by her side. The woman who answered the door is her daughter, Denise. Denise quietly shares with you that she thinks her mother may have had a stroke. You introduce yourself and your crew to Mrs. Messing. "Oh, everyone calls me Gloria," your patient replies. You notice her speech is comprehensible but slurred and slow. You quickly rule out any trauma. Todd says that Gloria had called him on the phone complaining of a headache and sounded odd. She was having a difficult time forming words and seemed to slur her speech slightly. He immediately called 9-1-1 and drove to her house. He found Gloria sitting on the couch when he came in. It is clear to you that Gloria currently has an open airway. You complete a primary assessment **Table 1** and obtain a set of baseline vital signs **Table 2**.

Table 1	Primary Assessment Findings for Gloria
General impression	65-year-old woman with possible stroke.
Chief complaint	Headache.
Mechanism of injury/ nature of illness	No trauma. Rule out possible stroke.
Level of consciousness	Alert and oriented to person, place, day, time, and event.
Airway	Open and patent.
Breathing	Respirations are within normal limits, chest expansion is equal bilaterally, no evidence of previous chest/cardiac surgery. Lung sounds are clear. High-flow oxygen applied via a nonrebreathing mask (NRM).
Circulation	Radial pulses are strong and regular.
Life threats	Maintain level of consciousness and determine stroke onset.
Pupils	Pupils are equal, round, regular in size, and react properly to light (PEARRL).
Pertinent negatives	Patient denies chest pain or pressure. Patient denies vomiting or losing consciousness. Patient denies trauma. No diabetic history.
Interventions	Determine stroke onset, raise stroke alert, immediate transport to a stroke center, supportive care, monitor vital signs, watch for changes in status.
Glasgow coma scale (GCS)	Score: 15 (eye opening, 4; verbal response, 5; motor response, 6).

Table 2	Baseline Vital Signs for Gloria
Respirations	12 breaths/min and regular
Pulse	108 beats/min and irregular
Skin	Warm, pink, and dry
Blood pressure	180/96 mm Hg
Oxygen saturation	89% on room air

You obtain a SAMPLE history, including signs and symptoms, allergies, medications, pertinent past medical history, last oral intake, and events leading up to the illness or injury, from Denise and Todd **Table 3**.

Neurologic Emergencies

Table 3 — SAMPLE History for Gloria

Signs and symptoms	Sudden and severe onset of headache, inability to properly move left hand or leg, left side facial droop.
	Speech is slurred, but still comprehensible.
Allergies	No known drug allergies.
Medications	Atorvastatin (Lipitor), multivitamin.
Pertinent past medical history	High cholesterol and hypertension.
Last oral intake	Lunch about 6 hours ago.
Events leading up to the injury or illness	Drove home from work feeling fine.
	Got home and had a sudden onset of headache and inability to move left arm.

Question 2

In addition to performing a primary assessment on this patient, what other evaluation should be performed? Why?

Question 3

Aside from a possible stroke, what other medical condition(s) should you assess for and rule out?

Your driver, Paul, informs you that advanced life support (ALS) just pulled into the driveway. You perform the steps in the Cincinnati Prehospital Stroke Scale before moving Gloria to the ambulance Table 4.

Table 4 — Cincinnati Prehospital Stroke Scale Results for Gloria

Arm drift	Left arm pronator drift, right arm normal.
Facial droop	Left side of face droops, right side normal.
Speech	Slow and slurred but comprehensible and using correct words.

On the basis of your assessment findings, you are fairly certain that Gloria has had a stroke. Once in the back of the ambulance, ALS technician Terry has set up an IV bag and introduces himself to Gloria. The closest stroke center is approximately 20 miles away. Fortunately, rush hour traffic has passed and the roads are clear and dry.

Question 4

Would there be any value in calling the emergency department ahead of time to alert them of this patient? Why or why not?

Question 5

As the ALS technician is starting an IV on the patient, what responsibilities do you now have?

You have about a 25-minute commute to Parkview Hospital, so you have plenty of time to perform a secondary assessment on Gloria **Table 5**.

Table 5	Secondary Assessment Findings for Gloria
Level of consciousness	Patient is alert and oriented to person, place, day, and event, but is having increased difficulty answering questions.
Airway	Intact and patent.
Breathing	Rate is within normal limits; no difficulty breathing; no pain on inspiration; lung sounds are clear and equal bilaterally. High-flow oxygen still administered via NRM.
Circulation	Pulses present in both upper extremities, strong and regular. Skin is warm, dry, and flushed.
Head/neck	Patient is reporting severe headache. No other deformities, contusions, abrasions, punctures, penetrations, paradoxical motion in the chest, burns, tenderness, lacerations, or swelling (DCAP-BTLS) noted on head or neck.
Chest	No DCAP-BTLS noted to chest. Lung sounds are clear and equal bilaterally with full expansion.
Abdomen	Soft, nontender, no rigidity.
Pelvis/genitalia	Pelvis is intact, no deformities or pain on palpation. Patient denies pain to genitalia region, inspection is deferred.
Lower extremities	No DCAP-BTLS noted to lower extremities. Pulses present in both lower extremities. Movement and sensation are diminished to the left lower extremity. Pulse, movement, and sensation positive in right lower extremity.
Upper extremities	No DCAP-BTLS noted to upper extremities. Pulses present in both upper extremities. Movement and sensation is positive in upper right extremity. Movement and sensation are diminished in the upper left extremity.
Back/neck	No pain/discomfort or DCAP-BTLS noted to back and neck.
Pain	Patient rates her headache as a 10 on a scale of 1 to 10. Denies any other pain.
Glasgow coma scale (GCS)	Score: 15 (eye opening, 4; verbal response, 5; motor response, 6).

Neurologic Emergencies

As you get closer to Parkview Hospital, you observe that it is becoming increasingly more challenging for Gloria to communicate with you and your crew. While Gloria is still conscious and appears to understand what you are saying, she is having a great deal of difficulty speaking. You ask Sharon to obtain another set of vital signs Table 6. You also find that her GCS score has diminished to 13 (eye, 4; verbal, 3; motor, 6). Her left pupil is sluggish to respond, but her right pupil is equal, round, regular in size, and reacts properly to light.

Table 6	Second Set of Vital Signs for Gloria
Respirations	14 breaths/min and regular
Pulse	100 beats/min and irregular
Skin	Warm, dry, and flushed
Blood pressure	182/98 mm Hg
Oxygen saturation	98% with high-flow oxygen

Question 6

Is there any significance in the change of the GCS score? What is your concern?

Terry has called ahead to Parkview Hospital. On arrival you are greeted by the stroke team. They usher you in to the medical bay. Gloria's daughter is already at the hospital anxiously awaiting her mother's arrival. She asks how her mother is doing and you tell her she is stable but is not able to communicate as well now as she did earlier.

Question 7

What patient information do you want to be sure to share with the hospital staff?

You tell the emergency department staff the findings of the Cincinnati Prehospital Stroke Scale and the approximate time of onset of Gloria's signs and symptoms. You also share with the staff Gloria's GCS score, which started as a 15 and has deteriorated to a 13. After you transfer Gloria to the bed and gather your equipment, you wish the family well and head out to start your patient care report. Before you leave the hospital, one of the stroke team nurses tells you that Gloria has had a hemorrhagic stroke and is now in the intensive care unit. They will have to wait out the next 24 hours to see what happens. You thank her for the update and head out to the ambulance with Terry and Sharon.

Case Analysis

Question 1

What information would you go over with your trainee en route to this call? What can you tell her to expect for this type of patient?

If you are responsible for training a new EMT, it is helpful to review expectations for all calls. Clear expectations of the trainee, roles of the other crew members, and what to expect for each type of call, based on dispatch information, should be reviewed prior to arriving at the call. If your trainee has a clear understanding of what his or her responsibilities are, then he or she can participate more fully in the call with more expertise. Have your trainee recall the signs and symptoms of stroke (facial drooping on one side of the face, intense headache, weakness or paralysis on one side of the body, inability to speak clearly, change in personality, arm drift, loss of bladder or bowel function, decreased level of consciousness, pupils unequal in size, and loss of vision or double vision). It is important for your trainee to understand that communication with the patient may be challenging. In addition, you should review priorities for treating the potential stroke patient.

Question 2

In addition to performing a primary assessment on this patient, what other evaluation should be performed? Why?

In addition to your general patient assessment, you need to include a more detailed neurologic assessment. There are a few standard neurologic assessments available to use for possible stroke patients. They are the Cincinnati Prehospital Stroke Scale **Table 7** and the Los Angeles Prehospital Stroke Screen **Table 8**. Both of these stroke assessment tools are derivatives of the National Institutes of Health Stroke Scale. Studies show that if your patient presents with any one of the three symptoms on the Cincinnati Prehospital Stroke Scale, there is a 72% chance that she is having a stroke. The Los Angeles Prehospital Stroke Screen also rules out other causes of altered mental status. Either one of these two screening tools may be used to further assess your possible stroke patient. Check your local protocols to see if one assessment scale is preferred over another. Stroke scales are specific to stroke signs and symptoms.

Table 7 — The Cincinnati Prehospital Stroke Scale

Test	Normal	Abnormal
Facial Droop (Ask patient to show teeth or smile.)	Both sides of face move equally well.	One side of face does not move as well as other.
Arm Drift (Ask patient to close eyes and hold both arms out with palms up.)	Both arms move the same, or both arms do not move.	One arm does not move, or one arm drifts down compared with the other side.
Speech (Ask patient to say, "The sky is blue in Cincinnati.")	Patient uses correct words with no slurring.	Patient slurs words, uses inappropriate words, or is unable to speak.

Table 8   The Los Angeles Prehospital Stroke Screen

Criteria	Yes	Unknown	No
1. Age > 45 y			
2. History of seizures or epilepsy absent			
3. Symptoms < 24 h			
4. At baseline, patient is not wheelchair-bound or bedridden			
5. Blood glucose between 60 and 400 mg dL			
6. Obvious asymmetry (right versus left) in any of the following three exam categories (must be unilateral):			
	Equal	Right Weak	Left Weak
Facial smile/grimace		Droop	Droop
Grip		Weak grip / No grip	Weak grip / No grip
Arm strength		Drifts down / Falls rapidly	Drifts down / Falls rapidly

Interpretation: If criteria 1-6 are marked yes, the probability of a stroke is 97%.

Question 3

Aside from a possible stroke, what other medical condition(s) should you assess for and rule out?

There are many other medical problems that may mimic a stroke or cause altered mental status. Altered mental status can be caused from seizures, low blood glucose (hypoglycemia), alcohol intoxication, medication use or abuse, street drugs/illicit drugs, allergic reactions, head trauma, brain tumors, and tumors of the spine. Many states require you to check the blood glucose level of any patient presenting with an altered mental status. Check your local protocols for guidelines on this.

Question 4

Would there be any value in calling the emergency department ahead of time to alert them of this patient? Why or why not?

When you have determined that your patient is experiencing a stroke, the receiving hospital should be notified. Most states have designated stroke centers (hospitals that meet certain criteria to be designated as a hospital that can accommodate stroke patients from the emergency department through admission). The designation of stroke centers came about to help improve the delivery of care to patients with acute stroke **Table 9**.

Table 9	Stroke Center Criteria
Written care protocols	
Integrated emergency response team	
Availability of computed tomography (CT) scans and interpretation 24 hours a day	
Neurosurgery capabilities	
Intensive care unit	
Stroke registry	
Rapid laboratory testing	

Question 5

As your ALS technician is starting an IV on the patient, what responsibilities do you now have?

Your responsibilities as a basic life support (BLS) provider do not change just because ALS arrives. You should continue to provide BLS care, including further assessing your patient. You may be asked to assist the ALS provider in getting, for example, an IV bag out to be hung. You will work together as a team to provide optimal patient care.

Question 6

Is there any significance in the change of the GCS score? What is your concern?

The GCS is used to determine and track the patient's neurologic status, such as level of alertness Table 10. Think of the GCS as a tool to help determine whether your patient is either deteriorating or improving. The patient's GCS should be assessed and recorded more than one time to help establish a trend in the patient's condition. The best score a patient can achieve is 15. The worst score would be 3. A GCS score of 13 indicates that the patient needs a timely transport to the nearest hospital for immediate definitive care.

Table 10 — Glasgow Coma Scale

Eye Opening		Best Verbal Response		Best Motor Response	
Spontaneous	4	Oriented conversation	5	Obeys commands	6
In response to speech	3	Confused conversation	4	Localizes pain	5
In response to pain	2	Inappropriate words	3	Withdraws to pain	4
None	1	Incomprehensible sounds	2	Abnormal flexion	3
		None	1	Abnormal extension	2
				None	1

Score: 13-15 may indicate mild dysfunction, although 15 is the score a person with no neurologic disabilities would receive.

Score: 9-12 may indicate moderate dysfunction.

Score: 8 or less is indicative of severe dysfunction.

Question 7

What patient information do you want to be sure to share with the hospital staff?

Proper transfer of the patient to the emergency department staff includes transferring all pertinent information, as well. Of particular importance in transferring patient information to the staff for a possible stroke patient is:

- Time of onset for stroke signs/symptoms
- Changes in level of consciousness
- GCS scores, including any changes to the GCS
- Stroke scale/score findings
- Any medical history pertinent to current condition (such as transient ischemic attacks, use of blood thinners, hypertensive medications, etc.)

Patient Care Report for Gloria

EMS Patient Care Report (PCR)

Date: 02-01-2010	Incident No.: 4521	Nature of Call: Possible stroke	Location: 1630 Westfall Road	
Dispatched: 1813	En Route: 1820	At Scene: 1827	Transport: 1839	At Hospital: 1904	In Service: 1919

Patient Information

Age: 65 years	Allergies: No known drug allergies
Sex: Female	Medications: Atorvastatin (Lipitor) and multivitamin
Weight (in kg [lb]): 86 kg (190 lb)	Past Medical History: High cholesterol and hypertension
	Chief Complaint: Headache

Vital Signs

Time	BP	Pulse	Respirations	SpO$_2$
1830	180/96	108 and irregular	12 and regular	93% on room air
1845	182/98	100 and irregular	14 and regular	98% with high-flow oxygen

EMS Treatment (circle all that apply)

Oxygen @ **15** L/min via (circle one): NC **(NRM)** Bag-mask Device

Assisted Ventilation	Airway Adjunct	CPR
Defibrillation	Bleeding Control	Bandaging	Splinting	Other:

Narrative

Responded to a call for a 65-year-old woman reporting severe and sudden onset of headache. Upon arrival at the single-family residence, patient found seated on the couch with family present. Patient was conscious and alert. Patient's daughter stated that she believes her mother may have had a stroke. Patient stated she went to work today and felt fine. Patient arrived home from work around 1800 hours when her head began to hurt. Patient also stated that at that time she was not able to move her left fingers. Patient made a phone call to a friend and her speech sounded slurred so the friend immediately called 9-1-1. Patient last ate lunch about 6 hours previous to incident. Patient denied any chest pain or pressure. Patient also denied losing consciousness and vomiting. Patient denied any injury or falls. Patient denied a history of diabetes. Medical history significant for hypertension and high cholesterol. Patient placed on high-flow oxygen and vital signs assessed. Cincinnati Prehospital Stroke Scale assessed and results were left arm pronator drift, right arm normal; left side facial droop, right side normal; speech was slow, deliberate, and correct words used without slurring. Initial GCS score is 15. Paramedic Terry met us on scene for ALS transport to Parkview Hospital. Secondary assessment was performed. Patient remained alert and oriented, but had increasing difficulty answering questions; airway remained intact; breathing rate was within normal limits with no difficulty breathing or pain noted; pulses present in both upper extremities, skin was warm and flushed; patient was complaining of a severe headache with 10/10 pain reported; no DCAP-BTLS noted anywhere on the body; abdomen was soft and nontender with no rigidity; pulse, movement, and sensation were present in lower right extremity, but diminished movement and sensation in lower left extremity; pulse, movement, and sensation were present in upper right extremity, but upper left extremity had diminished movement and sensation; no pain or discomfort noted to back or neck. Reassessment of GCS score is 13 (4/3/6). En route to Parkview Hospital, it was apparent that patient was having increased difficulty communicating with crew and speech was becoming increasingly slurred. Upon arrival at Parkview Hospital, crew and patient were greeted by the stroke team and ushered to the medical bay. Patient's daughter was waiting at hospital upon our arrival. Patient care transferred to emergency department neurologic staff. Bed rails raised, bed lowered. **End of report**

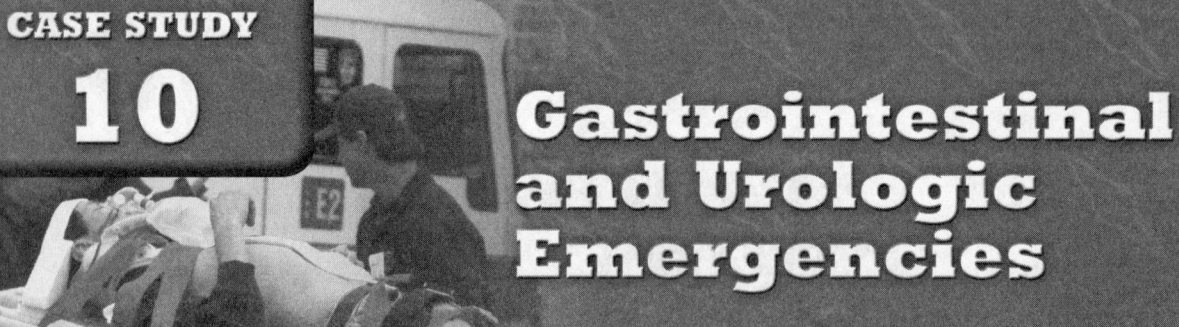

CASE STUDY 10

Gastrointestinal and Urologic Emergencies

Man With Back Pain and Nausea

It is early on a Saturday morning in San Antonio, Texas, when you hear the pager go off for a call at 6331 Cambridge Drive, Unit 4, for a 62-year-old man reporting back pain and nausea. You live close to the fire department where you work as an EMT, so you decide to respond to the call. You arrive at the firehouse to meet up with Bruce, who will drive the ambulance.

Time out of the firehouse is 0803.

You arrive at the apartment complex and find Unit 4 on the east end. You have been to these apartments before and are glad that there are no stairs to climb. As you approach the door you hear a dog barking and can see it jumping up in the front window.

"Please secure your dog so that we can enter," you yell through the front door.

After a minute, the dog is silent and the door opens. A woman ushers you inside where there is the pungent smell of tobacco smoke. Because you are carrying oxygen, you inquire if anybody is smoking. The woman assures you that no one is actively smoking. She is very worried about her brother, Reinardo. As she shows you to the back bedroom, she tells you that her brother called her earlier this morning to tell her he was not feeling well and asked if she could come over.

"He is a very proud man and is never sick. It is not like him to ask me to come over under such circumstances. When I arrived he looked so terrible. He was in his bed, very pale and moaning out in pain. He kept saying his back and stomach were hurting him. I did not know what else to do so I called 9-1-1," she says.

"You did the right thing by calling us, Ma'am," Bruce replies.

Question 1

Do you think you can get an idea of true urgency from this patient's sister or do you think she may be overreacting?

As you and Bruce enter the bedroom, you greet your patient and introduce yourself. Your patient acknowledges you and he tells you his name is Reinardo. He looks pale and in pain.

"My back and stomach ache and I feel like I am going to vomit," he says. Reinardo looks to be thin-to-medium build and of average weight for his size. He presents with an open airway and his breathing does not appear to be distressed. He gives you permission to assess him **Table 1** and obtain a set of baseline vital signs **Table 2**.

Table 1 — Primary Assessment Findings for Reinardo

General impression	62-year-old man complaining of back and abdominal pain.
Chief complaint	Severe pain to the lower back, groin, and abdomen.
Level of consciousness	Alert and oriented to person, place, day, time, and event.
Mechanism of injury/nature of illness	Abdominal and back pain.
Airway	Patent.
Breathing	Breathing is unlabored.
	Chest expansion is equal bilaterally.
	No trauma noted to the chest.
Circulation	Pulses are present in both upper extremities.
	No external bleeding noted.
	Skin is pale, clammy, and moist.
Life threats	Rule out acute abdomen, possible food poisoning, possible cardiac event, and musculoskeletal complaints.
Pupils	Pupils are equal, round, regular in size, and react properly to light (PEARRL).
Pertinent negatives	No trauma either today or recently.
Interventions	Oxygen 100% via nonrebreathing mask (NRM) applied due to unknown possible internal bleeding and to help alleviate nausea.
	Further assessment, treatment, and transport needed.
Pain	8 on a scale of 1 to 10.
Glasgow coma scale (GCS)	Score: 15 (eye opening, 4; verbal response, 5; motor response, 6).

Table 2 — Baseline Vital Signs for Reinardo

Respirations	22 breaths/min and shallow
Pulse	114 beats/min and irregular
Skin	Pale, clammy, and moist
Blood pressure	110/70 mm Hg
Oxygen saturation	96% on room air

Question 2

On the basis of your findings from the primary assessment, how would you prioritize this patient?

Question 3

What do you think is the best way to position the patient for transport?

Before moving Reinardo to the ambulance, you obtain a SAMPLE history, including signs and symptoms, allergies, medications, pertinent past medical history, last oral intake, and events leading up to the illness or injury Table 3.

Table 3 SAMPLE History for Reinardo

Signs and symptoms	Pain to lower back and abdomen. Pale, clammy, moist skin.
Allergies	No known drug allergies.
Medications	Aspirin for occasional aches and pains.
Pertinent past medical history	Chronic smoker for 40+ years; history of hypertension.
Last oral intake	Dinner last night at dinner time. No oral intake this morning.
Events leading up to the illness or injury	Awoke to use the bathroom at approximately 0600 hours when abdominal and back pain and nausea began.

Before you transfer Reinardo to the ambulance, his sister says, "He has not seen a doctor in quite some time. He has no insurance and no money for doctor's bills, so he has not gone in a few years. We know he has high blood pressure but he cannot afford the medications, so he does not take any right now."

You try your best to be reassuring to Reinardo's sister, Marcella, and thank her for the additional information. "Will you be riding with us to Southwest General Hospital or following in your own vehicle, Marcella?" Bruce asks.

"My daughter will give me a ride," she replies.

After securing the gurney in the ambulance, you tell Bruce to head toward Southwest General Hospital, which is approximately 18 miles away. "Reinardo, how are you feeling?" you ask.

"It hurts so much! Now it is starting to hurt down there, too!" He points to his groin area. You reassess his pain and he tells you it has increased to 9 on a scale of 1 to 10.

Question 4

Because your patient's pain has increased, what treatment and transport concerns do you have for him now?

You have a somewhat long commute to Southwest General; therefore, you have Bruce call for an advanced life support (ALS) rendezvous. ALS will meet up with you at a rest stop on the highway. Because Reinardo's pain has increased in intensity and has begun to radiate, you perform a secondary assessment Table 4.

Table 4	Secondary Assessment Findings for Reinardo
Level of consciousness	Patient is still conscious but in a great deal of pain and complaining of feeling light-headed. Patient's anxiousness is increasing as well.
Airway	Airway is patent.
Breathing	Lungs are clear with equal expansion bilaterally. Breathing is unlabored but shallow. Patient placed on high-flow oxygen because of increased pain and unknown possible internal bleeding. No trauma to the chest or surgical scars noted.
Circulation	Skin is now pale, warm, and dry. Peripheral pulses are absent now. Carotid pulse is present but weak and rapid. No external bleeding noted.
Head/neck	Pupils are sluggish to respond.
Chest	Unremarkable.
Abdomen	Distended and painful. Slight pulsating mass felt in the upper left abdominal quadrant.
Pelvis/genitalia	Painful genitalia, palpation not done, patient does not believe his genitalia are swollen, just painful.
Lower extremities	Movement and sensation are decreased in both lower extremities. Pulses are absent in both lower extremities. Patient's lower extremities are progressively becoming mottled and cyanotic.
Upper extremities	Movement and sensation are present in both upper extremities. Pulses are present in both upper extremities, but are weakening.
Back/neck	Increasing pain to the lower back area. No neck pain or trauma.
Pain	9 on a scale of 1 to 10.
Glasgow coma scale (GCS)	Score: 13 (eye opening, 3; verbal response, 4; motor response, 6).

You also collect a second set of vital signs for Reinaldo Table 5.

Table 5	Second Set of Vital Signs for Reinardo
Respirations	26 breaths/min, rapid and shallow
Pulse	120 beats/min, rapid and weak centrally (absent peripherally)
Skin	Pale, warm, and dry
Blood pressure	56/40 mm Hg
Oxygen saturation	96% on oxygen

Gastrointestinal and Urologic Emergencies

Question 5

What is a likely cause of this patient's change in vital signs?

"Ah! It hurts!" Reinardo cries out. He then stops talking. You reassess his airway, breathing, and circulation and find them still intact. You are relieved to know that ALS will be boarding your ambulance in less than a minute.

When ALS arrives, you brief the medic, Jennifer, on Reinardo's history, assessment, and vital signs and tell Bruce to use lights and sirens on the way to the hospital. Reinardo is indeed still breathing, but he is less responsive now. Jennifer establishes two large-bore IVs and begins fluid replenishment while you assist ventilations with a bag-mask device. You both suspect Reinardo might be suffering from a ruptured abdominal aortic aneurysm (AAA). You assess one more set of vital signs Table 6.

Table 6 Third Set of Vital Signs for Reinardo

Respirations	32 breaths/min, rapid and shallow (ventilations assisted)
Pulse	124 beats/min, rapid and weak centrally (absent peripherally)
Skin	Pale, warm, and clammy
Blood pressure	58/40 mm Hg
Oxygen saturation	89% on oxygen

Question 6

What is the best way to treat the patient's shock at this time?

On arrival, the emergency department staff is waiting for you. As you continue to ventilate your patient, Bruce and the hospital staff help wheel Reinardo into the trauma bay. While you are transferring patient care, you and Jennifer share patient information with the staff. You also tell them that Reinardo's sister, Marcella, should be arriving soon.

You wash your hands and leave with your equipment. When you see Jennifer later at the station, she tells you that the emergency department staff confirmed your diagnosis of an AAA. The patient has been rushed to the operating room.

Question 7

What is an abdominal aortic aneurysm (AAA)?

Case Analysis

Question 1

Do you think you can get an idea of true urgency from this patient's sister or do you think she may be overreacting?

This patient's sister appears genuinely concerned. She realizes that her brother is not likely to call for help without a reason. This emergency call should be evaluated with the same level of professionalism and detail as any other emergency call.

Question 2

On the basis of your findings from the primary assessment, how would you prioritize this patient?

Because of the patient's pain level, this patient may be prioritized as unstable.

Question 3

What do you think is the best way to position the patient for transport?

When there is no trauma involved, patients experiencing abdominal pain should be transported in their position of comfort. Most times this will be either lying on their sides with the legs flexed (fetal position) or lying on their backs with their legs flexed. Flexing the lower extremities helps to take pressure off the lower abdominal muscles, therefore decreasing the tension and pain to the area.

Question 4

Because your patient's pain has increased, what treatment and transport concerns do you have for him now?

Keeping in mind that pain is a vital indicator of distress, an increase in this patient's pain level is cause for concern. This patient needs definitive care to determine his exact cause of pain. Also, be ready for changes to this patient's level of consciousness and perfusion status.

Question 5

What is a likely cause of this patient's change in vital signs?

The dramatic drop in blood pressure is cause for great concern. This most likely indicates some type of internal bleeding. You should be prepared to treat hypovolemic shock.

Question 6

What is the best way to treat the patient's shock at this time?

The treatment for shock is to keep your patient warm, continue to administer high-flow oxygen, monitor the airway and breathing, and be prepared for more aggressive respiratory support such as assisted ventilations with a bag-mask device. If a timely meet up with ALS is possible, this would be optimal for patient care because ALS can provide fluid replacement therapy.

Question 7

What is an abdominal aortic aneurysm (AAA)?

The aorta is the largest artery in the body, carrying oxygen-rich blood to all parts of the body. It is sometimes referred to as the great artery. The aorta lies anterior to the spine and passes through the chest region, where it is called the thoracic aorta. As it passes further down into the abdomen, it is then called the abdominal aorta. The abdominal aorta supplies the lower half of the body with oxygen-rich blood. Sometimes a section of the abdominal aorta can stretch over time. This is known as an abdominal aortic aneurysm. Many aortic aneurysms in their early stages do not present with any signs or symptoms. Here is what to look for when the aneurysm begins to show signs and symptoms:

- Severe and sudden pain in the lower back
- Severe and sudden pain in the abdomen
- Pulsing feeling in the abdomen
- Abdominal discoloration
- Pulsating masses
- Abdominal or pelvic rigidity
- Signs of shock
- Poor peripheral perfusion
- Groin pain
- Testicular pain in males
- Changes in level of consciousness
- Occasionally syncope (fainting)
- Anxiety
- Nausea/vomiting
- Diaphoresis
- Clammy skin
- Dry mouth, excessive thirst

Patients with a suspected abdominal aortic aneurysm need rapid transport to a facility that can assess, diagnose, and treat the AAA as soon as possible. Without definitive care, these patients will die.

Some facts about abdominal aortic aneurysms are as follows:

- A ruptured AAA is the 13th leading cause of death in the United States, causing an estimated 15,000 deaths per year.
- White males have the highest incidence of deaths from ruptured AAAs than any other population.
- AAA is most common between the ages of 65 and 75.

Some risk factors for AAA include the following:

- History of hypertension
- Male gender
- Obesity
- Immediate relative with history of AAA
- History of smoking
- History of a high cholesterol level

Patient Care Report for Reinardo

EMS Patient Care Report (PCR)

Date: 05-05-2010	Incident No.: 103521	Nature of Call: Back pain and nausea	Location: 6331 Cambridge Drive, Unit 4		
Dispatched: 0802	En Route: 0803	At Scene: 0810	Transport: 0822	At Hospital: 0851	In Service: 0910

Patient Information

Age: 62 years	Allergies: No known drug allergies
Sex: Male	Medications: Aspirin
Weight (in kg [lb]): 80 kg (175 lbs)	Past Medical History: Hypertension, smoking
	Chief Complaint: Lower back, groin, and abdominal pain

Vital Signs

Time: 0814	BP: 110/70	Pulse: 114 and irregular	Respirations: 22 and shallow	Spo$_2$: 96% on room air
Time: 0828	BP: 56/40	Pulse: 120, rapid and weak centrally	Respirations: 26 rapid and shallow	Spo$_2$: 96% on oxygen
Time: 0836	BP: 58/40	Pulse: 124, rapid and weak (absent peripherally)	Respirations: 32, shallow and rapid (ventilations assisted)	Spo$_2$: 89% on oxygen

EMS Treatment
(circle all that apply)

Oxygen @ <u>15</u> L/min via (circle one): NC **(NRM)** Bag-Mask Device	**(Assisted Ventilation)**	**(Airway Adjunct)** OPA	CPR
Defibrillation	Bleeding Control	Bandaging	Splinting	Other:

Narrative

Dispatched to residence of 62-year-old man complaining of nausea and back, abdominal, and groin pain. Crew greeted at door by patient's sister. Strong odor of tobacco smoke present. Crew assured no smoking at time of entry. Crew directed to the bedroom where patient was found lying in bed. Patient presented with open and patent airway and no apparent breathing difficulties. Patient was alert and oriented. Patient denied any falls or other trauma. Patient rated pain as 8/10 to the lower back, groin, and abdominal area. Patient had this pain for approximately 2 hours. Oxygen applied 100% via NRM. Patient admitted to a 40-year smoking history and hypertension. Patient last ate dinner last night. No oral intake this morning. Patient's sister stated that patient called her this morning not feeling well and asked her to come over. Patient's sister called 9-1-1. Patient denied having a history of abdominal pain and back pain. Once on board the ambulance, patient complained of increasing pain to the abdomen. Patient was still conscious but in more pain. Patient also complained of feeling light-headed. Airway remained patent. Lungs were clear with equal expansion. Breathing was unlabored but shallow. No trauma or scars noted to the chest. Skin was then pale, warm, and dry. Peripheral pulses were absent, carotid pulse was present but weak and rapid, no external bleeding noted. Head and chest were unremarkable on examination. Abdomen was distended and painful. A pulsating mass was felt in the upper left abdominal quadrant. Patient's genitalia were then painful; patient did not believe his genitalia were swollen. Movement and sensation were decreased in both lower extremities. Pulses were absent in both lower extremities. Patient's lower extremities were progressively becoming mottled and cyanotic. Movement and sensation was present in both upper extremities; pulses were present but weakening. Patient reported increasing pain to the lower back area. No neck pain or trauma. Pain was at 9/10 and his GCS score was 13. Medic 10 met with crew for ALS transport to Southwest General Hospital. Due to increasing respiratory rate and decreasing lung expansion, crew assisted patient's ventilations en route to hospital. On arrival at hospital, patient was triaged and transferred to the trauma bay, where the trauma team was awaiting his arrival. **End of report**

CASE STUDY 11

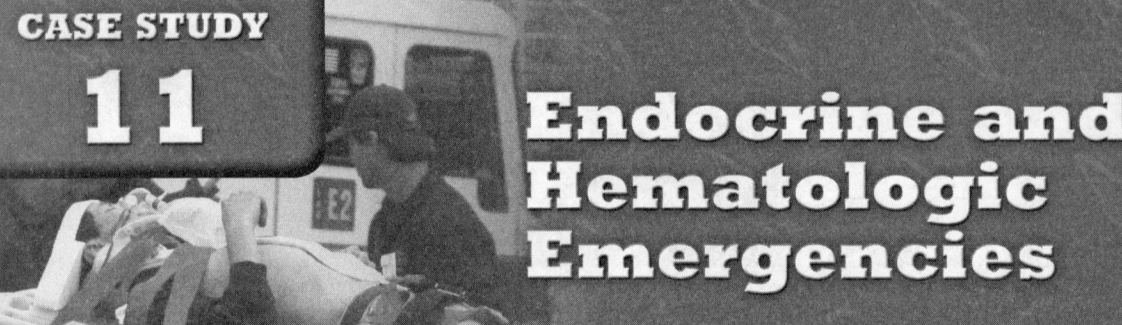

Endocrine and Hematologic Emergencies

Woman With a Possible Diabetic Reaction

It is a warm, sunny, August evening in Eugene, Oregon, when you and your partner, Larry, receive a call for a woman with a possible diabetic reaction in the pool at 22 West 14th Avenue. Since you have been an employee of the Eugene Ambulance Service for over 10 years, you are very familiar with the location. Time out is 1920.

You arrive on scene at 1926 hours and are greeted by one of the lifeguards, who escorts you to the stairs in the shallow end of the pool. A woman is sitting on the steps in the water next to her son. Another lifeguard is in the water in front of her. They tell you the woman's name is Faiza. She is 54 years old and is a diabetic.

You say hello to Faiza and she responds to you. Although her eyes are open, they are glassy and she does not appear to be able to follow (track) your movement very well. Her airway is patent and she is breathing normally.

Question 1

What might you ask the family and lifeguards about this patient?

You ask the lifeguards and the patient's son what happened to Faiza and how she got here. The lifeguard tells you that the patient was swimming in the deep end of the pool when she went over to the edge and just held on to the side looking confused. The lifeguard tried to talk with her to find out if anything was wrong. When she would not respond to him verbally, he got in the water and guided her to the steps. That is when the family came over to her and told the lifeguard that she is an insulin-dependent diabetic. The family then called 9-1-1. The son and the rest of the family are now with you near the patient.

Question 2

What other relevant questions about the patient's medical history should you ask the family at this point?

Her son informs you that the patient's last meal was about 5 or 6 hours ago. They also tell you that she forgot her blood glucose (BG) monitor at home in Vancouver, so she probably hasn't checked her sugar (glucose level) in a few days. The patient does not appear to be bleeding externally and does not seem to have sustained any trauma. Her radial pulse is slow, strong, and steady. Her skin is moist from being in the water and her forehead feels warm to the touch.

Question 3

How might you proceed with care for this patient?

You ask the lifeguard to assist you in getting Faiza out of the water. You both lead her to a nearby chair. The family wraps Faiza in some towels to keep her warm and dry her off.

Question 4

What are the steps in assessing a patient's blood glucose level?

Your partner Larry hands you the glucometer kit, which includes lancets, alcohol prep pads, sterile 2″ × 2″ gauze pads, and a few self-adhesive bandages. You obtain results in less than a minute. A finger stick reveals that Faiza's blood glucose level is 50 mg/dL.

With this information, you begin a primary assessment **Table 1**.

You obtain a SAMPLE history, including signs and symptoms, allergies, medications, pertinent past medical history, last oral intake, and events leading up to the illness or injury, from her family **Table 2**.

Table 1 Primary Assessment Findings for Faiza

General impression	54-year-old woman with altered level of consciousness.
Chief complaint	Altered mental status.
Level of consciousness	Alert but slow to respond to verbal stimuli.
Mechanism of injury/nature of illness	Altered mental status possibly due to hypoglycemia.
Airway	Patent.
Breathing	Breathing is unlabored. Chest expansion is equal bilaterally. No trauma noted to the chest.
Circulation	Pulses are present in both upper extremities. Skin is moist and warm. No external bleeding noted.
Life threats	Rule out acute abdomen, possible food poisoning, possible cardiac event, and musculoskeletal complaints.
Pupils	Pupils are equal, round, regular in size, and react properly to light (PEARRL).
Pertinent negatives	No trauma.
Glasgow coma scale (GCS)	Score: 14 (eye opening, 4; verbal response, 4; motor response, 6).

Table 2 SAMPLE History for Faiza

Signs and symptoms	Patient with altered mental status, conscious but not alert. No complaints of pain or discomfort.
Allergies	Sulfa drugs.
Medications	Insulin lispro (Humalog) 75/25 intramuscular, multivitamin, and vitamin E.
Pertinent past medical history	Insulin-dependent diabetes, mild neuropathy in the right lower extremity.
Last oral intake	Approximately 5 to 6 hours ago.
Events leading up to the illness or injury	Swimming in a pool at onset of hypoglycemia.

You ask the family if they have any orange juice or nondiet soda for Faiza to drink. They bring over a juice box and you encourage her to drink. She takes a sip and stares up at you. You and the family encourage her to drink more of the juice. She takes a few more sips but her mental status does not seem to be changing at this point. Larry suggests giving her some peanut butter crackers.

Faiza eats the crackers, and after finishing them, she looks at her family and asks, "What is going on?" Her family breathes a sigh of relief. Once they tell her what happened, Faiza smiles and laughs. You ask her if you can assess her blood glucose level again. She agrees and her numbers have improved. Her level is up to 81 mg/dL. She tells you that her normal blood glucose range is around 100 mg/dL.

You encourage Faiza to drink more of the juice and ask her if she would like to be transported to the hospital for evaluation. She declines and says that she will be fine now that she has had something to eat. She promises to be more careful for the duration of her visit. You ask her permission to assess her vital signs. She readily complies **Table 3**.

Table 3 Baseline Vital Signs for Faiza

Respirations	16 breaths/min and regular
Pulse	68 beats/min and regular
Skin	Warm, dry, and pale mucosa
Blood pressure	146/82 mm Hg
Oxygen saturation	99% on ambient air

Question 5

How should you respond when a patient refuses treatment/transport?

Question 6

What questions should be addressed before a patient is allowed to sign an official release form?

After you determine that Faiza is alert and oriented and has no complaints, she signs the refusal of treatment. Although she has refused treatment, you ask her if you may assess her vitals one more time to confirm her condition has improved. She agrees **Table 4**. Her son, Sanjib, signs as a witness. You give her a copy of the Health Insurance Portability and Accountability Act (HIPAA) policies and wish her well, reminding her that she can call 9-1-1 again if her condition changes.

Table 4	Second Set of Vital Signs for Faiza
Respirations	12 breaths/min and regular
Pulse	68 beats/min and regular
Skin	Warm, dry, and pink mucosa
Blood pressure	140/80 mm Hg
Oxygen saturation	100% on ambient air

Case Analysis

■ Question 1

What might you ask the family and lifeguards about this patient?

Asking the lifeguards and family members what happened to this patient is a good place to start. You should also ask about the patient's normal behavior and how her behavior changes in an insulin emergency. You should immediately inquire as to whether the patient sustained any trauma or loss of consciousness in the pool.

■ Question 2

What other relevant questions about the patient's medical history should you ask the family at this point?

The following questions may be asked:
- Has she eaten normally today?
- When did she last check her sugar levels?
- What does she prefer to eat to raise her sugar levels?
- Has she ever lost consciousness because of her diabetes?
- Has she taken her usual dose of insulin today?
- Has she taken any other medications today?
- Does she comply with her medication regimen(s)?
- Has she had any unusual stress today?
- Does she see her doctor regularly?

If the son hadn't already indicated so, you should also ask whether Faiza is dependent on insulin to manage her diabetes.

■ Question 3

How might you proceed with care for this patient?

Once you have ruled out any trauma, it would be advisable to assist the patient out of the water immediately. Despite the warm weather, her altered level of consciousness raises the concern that she could become hypothermic in the water. Be sure to dry her off when she is out of the water to help preserve her body temperature.

Question 4

What are the steps in assessing a patient's blood glucose level?

Before you can assess a patient's blood glucose level, you must first have the proper supplies, which include the following:
- Body substance isolation/personal protective equipment
- Alcohol pads
- Safety lancets
- Sharps container
- Glucometer
- Chemistry strips
- Sterile 2″ × 2″ gauze pads
- Self-adhesive bandages

Once you have the correct supplies, follow these steps to assess a blood glucose level:
- Talk to your patient and explain what you are doing.
- Prepare the glucometer.
- The site may be massaged or warmed prior to cleaning to assist in increasing blood flow to the area.
- Use an alcohol pad to clean the fingertip that you are going to prick with the lancet.
- Wrap your fingers around the patient's finger with your non-dominant hand at the base of the patient's nail bed, test site up. This will give you control over the patient's finger while performing the finger stick.
- Press the lancet against the skin firmly.
- The first drop of blood should be wiped off onto a sterile 2″ × 2″ gauze pad.
- The second drop of blood should then be placed on the tip of the test strip. (Some glucometers draw up blood into the test strip automatically.)
- The glucometer will give you a reading in about 3 to 10 seconds.
- While awaiting test results of the blood glucose test, place a sterile gauze pad over the site and apply gentle pressure to stop any bleeding.
- Record the number from the glucometer into your documentation.
- Cover the test site with a sterile self-adhesive bandage as needed.

Question 5

How should you respond when a patient refuses treatment/transport?

When transport is refused, you must assess whether the patient is able to make an informed decision. Because the patient has experienced an altered mental status and had not checked her blood glucose level in a few days, explain to her that it is important for her to receive further evaluation at the hospital. Although her vital signs were stable and her glucose level has increased, the level has not been raised to her normal range of approximately 100 mg/dL. Make every effort to encourage the patient to permit transport and continued treatment. That being said, however, a competent adult does have the right to refuse treatment and/or transport.

Question 6

What questions should be addressed before a patient is allowed to sign an official release form?

When the patient refuses care and wants to sign a refusal form, you must fully document the refusal. Documentation should include any assessment findings that you were able to make, your efforts to obtain consent, and the patient's signature as witnessed by a family member or law enforcement officer.

The following questions should be addressed when a patient refuses treatment/transport:
- Is the patient oriented to person, place, time, day, and event?
- Has the patient sustained any head injury or trauma?
- Is there a possibility of drug or alcohol use?
- Is the patient a minor? (Check the age at which a person is no longer considered a minor in your state.)
- Is there any evidence that the patient is a threat to himself or herself or others?

The following checklist can be used when a patient refuses treatment/transport:
- Determine that the patient has the capacity to refuse treatment/transport.
- Explain the risks of refusing treatment/transport.
- Confirm that the patient understands your explanation.
- Encourage the patient to seek further medical treatment from a personal physician or by calling 9-1-1.
- Obtain the patient's signature on a refusal form and the signature of a responsible witness.

Patient Care Report for Faiza

EMS Patient Care Report (PCR)

Date: 08-23-10	Incident No.: 11255	Nature of Call: Diabetic emergency	Location: 22 West 14th Avenue	
Dispatched: 1918	En Route: 1920	At Scene: 1926	Transport:	At Hospital:	In Service: 1951

Patient Information

Age: 54 years	**Allergies:** Sulfa drugs
Sex: Female	**Medications:** Insulin lispro (Humalog) 75/25 intramuscular, multivitamin, and vitamin E
Weight (in kg [lb]): 73 kg (160 lb)	**Past Medical History:** Insulin-dependent diabetes, mild neuropathy in the right lower extremity
	Chief Complaint: Altered mental status

Vital Signs

Time	BP	Pulse	Respirations	SpO$_2$
1930	146/82	68 and regular	16 and regular	99% on ambient air
1940	140/80	68 and regular	12 and regular	100% on ambient air

EMS Treatment (circle all that apply)

Oxygen @ **15** L/min via (circle one): NC NRM Bag-Mask Device	Assisted Ventilation	Airway Adjunct	CPR
Defibrillation	Bleeding Control	Bandaging	Splinting	**(Other:)** Assessed BG level

Narrative

Dispatched to apartment complex pool for a 54-year-old woman having a possible diabetic reaction. Patient found seated on steps of pool, attended to by lifeguard. Patient's airway was open with no obvious obstructions. Breathing did not appear to be labored. The lifeguard explained that the patient was swimming in the deep end when she became disoriented. The lifeguard got into the pool and guided the patient from the deep end to the steps, where they awaited the ambulance crew. Lifeguard and family denied any trauma to the patient. Patient's initial GCS was 14. Patient's son was present on the deck of the pool and told emergency medical services (EMS) crew that patient is an insulin-dependent diabetic. Patient last ate about 5-6 hours prior. Unknown when patient last checked her blood glucose as she is visiting from Vancouver, Canada, and forgot to bring her glucometer with her. Lifeguard assisted in getting the patient out of the water and into a chair on deck. Family members wrapped patient with dry towels. Blood glucose level assessed at 50 mg/dL. Patient given juice to drink but this did not have effect on level of consciousness. Patient also given peanut butter crackers, which increased her level of consciousness. Patient was then alert. Repeat glucose level measured at 81 mg/dL. Patient's normal level is about 100 mg/dL. Patient finished the juice and refused transport, but did allow crew to assess vital signs as noted above. Patient's GCS increased to 15 after she ate peanut butter crackers. Patient was alert and oriented and had no complaints. Patient signed release form and patient's son signed as a witness. Patient was encouraged to call 9-1-1 again if needed. No further treatment, no transport. **End of report**

CASE STUDY 12

Toxicology

Intoxicated Man

The pager sounds and bells in the firehouse wake you out of a deep sleep. The clock reads 0335 hours. Your partner, Tyler, groans as you get up and answer the call. The dispatcher gives the following information: "Ambulance requested at the corner of Orange Avenue and 7th Street for an intoxicated man lying on the ground, moaning."

"BLS 2559 responding from quarters," you reply.

You arrive on the scene to find a man in his 50s lying on the sidewalk in a left lateral recumbent position. A well-worn bicycle is on its side next to him. His clothes are visibly soiled and his hair is very unkempt. The two police officers on the scene tell you that they have seen him frequently intoxicated. You ask if there were any witnesses as to how he got here. The police officers say there was no one around when they found him.

Question 1

What special concerns might you have for any call involving an intoxicated person?

Question 2

Which signs and symptoms would you expect an intoxicated person to exhibit on a call?

Question 3

What type of approach should you take with this patient? Should you treat this as a trauma scene, a medical scene, or both? Why?

You introduce yourself and your partner to the patient and inquire about what is bothering him. Tyler gently maintains head stabilization. Your patient shows no objection to Tyler touching him and answers your questions. He tells you that his name is Jim and that nothing is bothering him, other than he is cold and thirsty.

Question 4

Can you get a reliable patient history from an intoxicated patient?

"Jim, have you been drinking this evening?" you ask.

He replies, "Yup!"

"How much do you think you had to drink?" you ask.

"I can't remember, I've been drinking all day to keep warm," Jim says. With Tyler holding head stabilization, you tell Jim you are going to roll him over on his back. The patient denies having any pain. Now that he is in a supine position, it is much easier to assess him. He complies readily with the primary assessment **Table 1** and SAMPLE history, including signs and symptoms, allergies, medications, pertinent past medical history, last oral intake, and events leading up to the illness or injury **Table 2**. You also obtain a set of baseline vital signs **Table 3**.

Table 1 — Primary Assessment Findings for Jim

General impression	53-year-old intoxicated man, complaining of back and abdominal pain.
Chief complaint	Abdominal pain and low back pain.
Mechanism of injury/nature of illness	Alcohol ingestion and possible fall off bicycle.
Level of consciousness	Alert to person and location, not aware of time of day or day of the week.
Airway	Patent.
Breathing	Breathing is unlabored. Chest expansion is equal bilaterally. No trauma to the chest. Oxygen applied due to unknown possible internal bleeding.
Circulation	Pulses present in both upper extremities. No external bleeding.
Life threats	Rule out back injury and abdominal pain.
Pertinent negatives	No complaints of chest pain/discomfort, denies shortness of breath, denies pain anywhere other than his low back and abdomen. Unsure if he lost consciousness.
Pupils	Slow to react bilaterally.
Interventions	Oxygen administered. Further assessment, treatment, and transport needed.
Pain	Patient is unable to determine level of pain.
Glasgow coma scale (GCS)	Score: 14 (eye opening, 4; verbal response, 4; motor response, 6).

Table 2 — SAMPLE History for Jim

Signs and symptoms	Possible alcohol intoxication, patient complaining of back and abdominal pain, plus thirst and feeling cold.
Allergies	Unknown.
Medications	None currently.
Pertinent past medical history	Unknown; patient cannot remember.
Last oral intake	Patient admits to drinking beer 2 hours ago. Cannot remember last time he ate.
Events leading up to the injury or illness	He thinks he may have just come out of the convenience store when he laid down on the side walk to rest. No witnesses as to how he got on the sidewalk.

Table 3 — Baseline Vital Signs for Jim

Respirations	12 breaths/min, shallow and regular
Pulse	72 beats/min and regular
Skin	Warm, flushed, and dry
Blood pressure	156/78 mm Hg
Oxygen saturation	98% on ambient air

You and Tyler immobilize the patient on a backboard and move him to the warmth of the ambulance. You inform Jim that you will take him to Sharp Coronado Hospital for further evaluation. About 10 minutes from the emergency department, Jim vomits. You can see bright red blood in his vomitus and it smells of alcohol. After you suction out his mouth, Jim says, "I want to get off this board! It's so uncomfortable!" You assure him that when you get to the hospital he will be taken off the board by the hospital staff. You complete another set of vital signs Table 4 and a secondary assessment Table 5.

Table 4 — Second Set of Vital Signs for Jim

Respirations	12 breaths/min, full and regular
Pulse	70 beats/min and regular
Skin	Warm, flushed, and dry
Blood pressure	154/76 mm Hg
Oxygen saturation	100% on high-flow oxygen

Toxicology

Table 5 Secondary Assessment Findings for Jim

Level of consciousness	Alert and oriented now to person, place, and day of the week.
Airway	Patent.
Breathing	Breathing is still unlabored.
	Chest expansion is equal bilaterally.
	No deformities, contusions, abrasions, punctures, penetrations, paradoxical movement of the chest, bruises, tenderness, lacerations, or swelling (DCAP-BTLS) noted to the chest.
	Oxygen applied due to internal bleeding.
Circulation	Pulses strong and regular.
	No external bleeding noted.
	Skin is still warm, dry, and flushed to the face.
Head/neck	No pain or injuries noted to head or neck.
	Cervical collar applied.
	Pupils are slow to react bilaterally.
Chest	Lung sounds clear and equal bilaterally with equal expansion.
	No DCAP-BTLS to chest.
Abdomen	Distended; tender but not rigid.
	No bruising or scarring noted to abdomen.
Pelvis/genitalia	Pelvis intact, no complaints of genitalia pain/discomfort so genitalia exam deferred.
Lower extremities	Pulse, movement, and sensation positive in both lower extremities.
	Bruising noted to right lower extremity in the tibia/fibula area, but no swelling.
Upper extremities	Pulse, movement, and sensation positive in both upper extremities.
	No DCAP-BTLS noted.
Back/neck	Tenderness to lower back, otherwise unremarkable.
Pain	Patient states his lower back hurts and now can articulate a pain level of 3 on a scale of 1 to 10.
	Pain to abdomen is 6 on a scale of 1 to 10.
Glasgow coma scale (GCS)	Score: 15 (eye opening, 4; verbal response, 5; motor response, 6).

After you complete a secondary assessment, you ask Jim for some demographic information. He tells you he has a "benefit" card, but that he does not have an address or phone number.

Question 5

Apart from the patient's medical information that you would share with the triage nurse, what other pertinent information might you consider sharing?

Question 6

While en route to a hospital, if a patient decides that he or she no longer wants treatment and does not want to go to the hospital, can you allow him or her to sign a release and leave? Why or why not?

At triage, you tell the nurse Jim's medical history and indicate that he appears to be homeless. The emergency department has a record for Jim because he has been there before. Prior to moving him to a trauma bed, the triage nurse obtains a blood alcohol level on Jim using a breathalyzer. It registers 0.28. You and Tyler transfer him to bed 12 in the trauma bay, cover him with a warm hospital blanket, lower the bed to the lowest position, put the side rails up on the bed, and relay information to the nurse who will be caring for him.

Case Analysis

■ Question 1

What special concerns might you have for any call involving an intoxicated person?

As with any call, scene safety is a priority. Patients who are intoxicated from alcohol or other drugs may respond to EMS providers irrationally or violently. Caution should be used and you should not to let your guard down with patients under the influence of drugs or alcohol.

■ Question 2

Which signs and symptoms would you expect an intoxicated person to exhibit on a call?

Signs and symptoms of intoxicated patients may be similar to those of persons who are not intoxicated. Patients under the effects of alcohol, however, oftentimes have a diminished sense of pain. They also may present with a depressed respiratory drive, depending on how intoxicated they are and their normal tolerance for alcohol. Large motor movements may be depressed as well.

■ Question 3

What type of approach should you take with this patient? Should you treat this as a trauma scene, a medical scene, or both? Why?

Until proven otherwise, this patient should be treated as both a trauma patient and a medical patient. In this scenario, which came first, the fall or the illness? Did this patient fall because he was suffering a medical emergency or did this patient sustain trauma first and then experience a medical problem after the fall?

■ Question 4

Can you get a reliable patient history from an intoxicated patient?

It is challenging to ascertain a reliable medical history from an intoxicated patient because of the patient's altered mental status and the effects of the alcohol in his or her system. Again, these patients frequently have a diminished sense of pain when they are under the influence. Their sense of time (onset, events leading up to the event, etc.) may be inaccurate as well.

■ Question 5

Apart from the patient's medical information that you would share with the triage nurse, what other pertinent information might you consider sharing?

Where and how this patient was found are valuable clues to his situation. If Jim is homeless, the staff at the hospital can attempt to contact services for Jim to try to better his circumstances. Also, telling the triage nurse that Jim is homeless can indicate that he most likely does not seek medical care on a regular basis. He may not be up to date with his vaccinations.

■ Question 6

While en route to a hospital, if a patient decides that he or she no longer wants treatment and does not want to go to the hospital, can you allow him or her to sign a release and leave? Why or why not?

All competent adult patients have the right to refuse care at any time. When treatment is refused, you must assess the patient's ability to make an informed decision. If a patient appears confused, he or she cannot legally decline care. When in doubt, always act in the best medical interest of the patient. Again, think critically here. What could happen to this patient if he were released from your treatment? Some things that may help convince a patient that continued care is in his or her best interest would include telling the patient you care about his or her well-being and that you are concerned.

Patient Care Report for Jim

EMS Patient Care Report (PCR)			
Date: 01-21-2011	**Incident No.:** 20112578	**Nature of Call:** Intoxicated patient	**Location:** Orange Avenue and 7th Street
Dispatched: 0335	**En Route:** 0338	**At Scene:** 0346 / **Transport:** 0404	**At Hospital:** 0417 / **In Service:** 0443

Patient Information

Age: 53 years	**Allergies:** Unknown
Sex: Male	**Medications:** None
Weight (in kg [lb]): 86 kg (190 lb)	**Past Medical History:** Unknown
	Chief Complaint: Low back and abdominal pain

Vital Signs

Time	BP	Pulse	Respirations	SpO$_2$
0352	156/78	72 and regular	12 shallow and regular	98% on ambient air
0405	154/76	70 and regular	12 full and regular	100% on high-flow oxygen

EMS Treatment (circle all that apply)

Oxygen @ **15** L/min via (circle one): NC **(NRM)** Bag-mask Device	Assisted Ventilation	Airway Adjunct	CPR
Defibrillation	Bleeding Control	Bandaging	Splinting	**(Other:)** spinal immobilization, oral suctioning

Narrative

Dispatched to a call for an intoxicated man on the sidewalk of Orange Avenue. On arrival patient found lying in the left lateral recumbent position on the sidewalk, with his bike lying next to him. There were two law enforcement officers present. The officers on scene stated that they are familiar with this patient. They were not witnesses as to how the patient got on the sidewalk. Head stabilized by Tyler on initial contact with patient. Patient complained of being cold and thirsty. Patient admitted to drinking alcohol earlier in the evening and stated he was "drinking all day to keep warm." Patient denied any pain at that point, and was rolled over to a supine position. Patient was alert to person and location, but not to day and time. Patient's airway was patent with no obstructions. Breathing was unlabored with equal chest expansion. High-flow oxygen administered via nonrebreathing mask. Chest was negative for trauma. Pulses were present in both upper extremities, no external bleeding noted. Skin was warm, flushed, and dry. Patient complained of abdominal and lower back pain but was unable to determine pain level. Patient denied any medications and could not remember a medical history or any allergies. Patient could not remember the last time he ate. As we gathered further history, patient believed he was coming out of the convenience store when he laid down on the sidewalk to rest. Patient denied any chest pain or discomfort, shortness of breath, or pain anywhere other than his low back and abdomen. Patient could not remember if he lost consciousness. Patient moved to ambulance via a long board with full spinal immobilization via cervical collar. Patient vomited en route to hospital. Vomitus contained bright red blood and smelled of alcohol. Patient's airway was suctioned. Secondary assessment was performed. Patient was alert and oriented to person, place, and day. Airway was patent; breathing remained unlabored with equal chest expansion. No DCAP-BTLS noted to the chest. Oxygen remained in place via a nonrebreathing mask. Pulses were strong and regular, no external bleeding was noted anywhere. Skin remained warm, dry, and flushed to the face. No pain or injuries noted to the head or neck. Lung sounds were clear bilaterally. Abdomen was distended and diffusely tender, but not rigid. No bruising or scarring noted to abdomen. Pelvis was intact, no complaints of genitalia pain, genitalia exam deferred. Pulse, movement, and sensation are positive in both lower extremities. Bruising was noted to the right lower extremity in the tibia/fibula area, but no swelling. Pulse, movement, and sensation were positive in both upper extremities. No DCAP-BTLS noted to upper extremities. Tenderness to the lower back, otherwise unremarkable. Patient stated his lower back hurt and articulated a pain level of 3/10. GCS score improved to 15 (4/5/6). Patient triaged and moved to the trauma bay. Patient covered with blankets; bed rails up, bed lowered to lowest position. Patient left in the care of hospital staff. **End of report**

CASE STUDY 13

Psychiatric Emergencies

Teenage Girl With Forearm Lacerations

It has been a long shift and you and your partner are happy that the day is almost over. You then feel your pager vibrate and hear the tones sound. You have one more call to take before you can call it a day. It is 2234 hours and you are being dispatched to a call for a teenage girl who has cut herself. Police are on the scene and will advise you when it is safe to enter. You are asked to stage several blocks away. You and your driver, Duncan, head to the safe staging location and consider the possibilities of this call. Law enforcement calls you into the scene at approximately 2246 hours. One of the police officers flags you in through the front door of the single-family residence.

Question 1

What approach would you use to ensure your safety and that of your partner on this call?

Your patient, Christina, is 13 years old. She is sitting quietly on the couch in the living room with her head down and her hands in the pockets of her baggy, hooded sweatshirt. Her airway is intact and breathing appears adequate. There are three police officers on the scene—two of them are with the patient in the living room. They tell you that Christina was angry with her mother and decided to cut herself on the wrists. Christina has admitted that she and a group of classmates frequently engage in similar behavior. What prompted the 9-1-1 call this evening, however, was the fact that she had cut herself deeper than normal and was afraid she had cut too far.

You introduce yourself to Christina and ask her how she is feeling. She tells you that her left wrist hurts and she is a bit embarrassed by all the attention. You note bilateral chest rise and good air exchange. You then assess her wrists and find several horizontal incisions there. The cuts on her left wrist appear as though they will need sutures. Law enforcement tells you that they have contacted Christina's mother and she will meet you at St. Mary's Hospital. They also tell you that Christina is being placed on a psychiatric hold until pending evaluation at the hospital. There are no other related adults, friends, or family members in the home at this time. You perform a primary assessment **Table 1** and obtain a set of baseline vital signs **Table 2**.

Table 1 — Primary Assessment Findings for Christina

General impression	Called to transport a patient (13-year-old girl) on a psychiatric hold by law enforcement.
Chief complaint	Wrist pain from lacerations.
Level of consciousness	Alert and oriented to person, place, time, and event.
Airway	Patent.
Breathing	Breathing is unlabored. Chest expansion is equal bilaterally. No trauma noted to the chest. Lung sounds are clear.
Circulation	Pulses present in both upper extremities. Bleeding from wrist lacerations on left wrist.
Life threats	External hemorrhage from wrist lacerations, risk of threat to self and/or others.
Pupils	Pupils are equal, round, regular in size, and react properly to light (PEARRL).
Interventions	Sterile gauze placed over wounds. Further assessment, treatment, and transport needed.
Pain	4 on a scale of 1 to 10.
Glasgow coma scale (GCS)	Score: 15 (eye opening, 4; verbal response, 5; motor response, 6).

Table 2 — Baseline Vital Signs for Christina

Respirations	18, regular and unlabored
Pulse	98 and regular
Skin	Pink, warm, and dry
Blood pressure	122/90 mm Hg
Oxygen saturation	100% on room air

Question 2

Does this patient have the potential to become violent?

The patient is being cooperative, so you decide to obtain SAMPLE history before transport, including signs and symptoms, allergies, medications, pertinent past medical history, last oral intake, and events leading up to the illness or injury **Table 3**.

Table 3   SAMPLE History for Christina

Signs and symptoms	Wrist pain due to self-inflicted lacerations
Allergies	No known allergies to medications
Medications	Ibuprofen, as needed (PRN)
Pertinent past medical history	None
Last oral intake	Pizza and soda around 2200 hours
Events leading up to the injury or illness	Angry with mom, so decided to cut wrists in protest

As you are gathering information from the police officers, your partner applies 100% oxygen via a nonrebreathing mask and places sterile gauze over the injured areas to minimize infection risks. You inquire about what she used to cut herself with. The police believe it was a razor blade, but they have not located it. The razor blade could be used as a weapon, so caution must be taken until it is located. Eventually, the razor blade is found in Christina's bedroom and the police officers have searched Christina for any other possible weapons.

Christina is brought to the ambulance for transport to St. Mary's Hospital emergency department. Because she is secured to the gurney with the seat belts and shoulder harness, you do not need police detail in the ambulance, and therefore a police officer will follow you to the hospital. Christina is quiet but cooperative en route to the hospital.

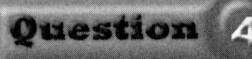

Question 3

In addition to your regular SAMPLE history, what other questions might you ask to help assess this situation and patient?

On your arrival at the hospital, the triage nurse, Sarah, takes in all the patient information and sends you back to bed 6 in the pediatric trauma bay. Christina must first be cleared medically before she can be moved to the psychiatric floor for an evaluation. You transfer Christina to bed 6 in the trauma bay of the pediatric emergency department without any incident.

Question 4

What are some legal considerations for the treatment and transport of this patient?

Case Analysis

■ Question 1

What approach would you use to ensure your safety and that of your partner on this call?

Staging until law enforcement has cleared the scene is the recommended approach to take.

■ Question 2

Does this patient have the potential to become violent?

First, never assume that a teenage girl does not have potential to harm you. Undoubtedly, the answer here is "yes." Once inside the scene, even with police presence, caution should be used on calls like this. Do not assume someone else will be responsible for your safety. Be aware that any person, child or adult, if under the influence of substances or psychologically unstable, is a potential threat to you. You also do not know whether drugs or alcohol are involved. Sometimes patients under the influence of drugs or alcohol have lowered inhibitions, increased physical strength, and may even become violent.

■ Question 3

In addition to your regular SAMPLE history, what other questions might you ask to help assess this situation and patient?

Table 4 Lists questions that may help you evaluate a patient with a mental health disorder.

Table 4 — Questions to Ask in Evaluating a Mental Health Disorder

- Does the patient answer your questions appropriately?
- Does the patient's behavior seem appropriate?
- Does the patient seem to understand you and the surroundings?
- Is the patient withdrawn or detached? Hostile or friendly? Elated or depressed?
- Are the patient's vocabulary and expressions what you would expect under the circumstances?
- Does the patient seem aggressive or dangerous to you or others?
- Is the patient's memory intact? Check orientation to time, place, person, and event: What day, month, and year is it? Who am I?
- Does the patient express disordered thoughts, delusions, or hallucinations?

Question 4

What are some legal considerations for the treatment and transport of this patient?

Because this patient is a minor, special consent needs to be taken into consideration. The patient's parent or guardian is not available to obtain consent. However, because this patient is in police custody, the police can assume legal responsibility for the patient. Many states have some form of a psychiatric hold law or a mental hygiene (mental illness) arrest law. A psychiatric hold allows police officers to take at-risk patients into custody to seek out entry into mental health treatment. At-risk patients may be those who exhibit behavior that would be considered violent towards self or others, for example. If these patients are not willing to seek treatment themselves, then law enforcement officers can legally take them into custody to do so. Because law enforcement officers oftentimes play a fundamental role in entry into mental health services and are a common source of referral to psychiatric emergency care, there are laws that govern how police officers may assist such patients in reaching the care they may desperately need. Many times law enforcement and EMS personnel come across such people when responding to EMS calls for service such as "possible suicide," or other behavioral emergency crisis. Another consideration to keep in mind is that you are transporting a teenage female patient. Whenever possible, it would be ideal to have a female provider in the back of the rig with her. Accusations of inappropriate behavior are less likely to occur if a same-sex provider is with this patient. Follow up with thorough documentation. Be sure to include where the patient was located during transport, where you sat during transport, any pertinent conversation that took place, what clothes and belongings the patient was transported with, mileage from the residence to the hospital, times of the call (including time to triage and time to hospital bed), and in whose care the patient was left.

Patient Care Report for Christina

EMS Patient Care Report (PCR)

Date: 01-12-2011	Incident No.: 2245	Nature of Call: Cut/5150		Location: 125 Greenvale Drive	
Dispatched: 2234	En Route: 2236	At Scene: 2246	Transport: 2259	At Hospital: 2314	In Service: 2335

Patient Information

Age: 13 years	Allergies: No known drug allergies
Sex: Female	Medications: Ibuprofen prn
Weight (in kg [lb]): 66 kg (145 lb)	Past Medical History: None
	Chief Complaint: Pain to left wrist

Vital Signs

Time	BP	Pulse	Respirations	SpO₂
2256	122/90	98 and regular	18 and regular	100% on oxygen

EMS Treatment (circle all that apply)

Oxygen @ **15** L/min via (circle one): NC **(NRM)** Bag-valve device		Assisted Ventilation	Airway Adjunct	CPR
Defibrillation	Bleeding Control	**(Bandaging)**	Splinting	Other:

Narrative

Dispatched to a call for a 13-year-old girl who allegedly cut her wrist. After staging, called into scene by the Brighton Police Department at approximately 2246 hours. On arrival, patient found seated on the living room couch, with three police officers present. Patient's airway intact and breathing appeared adequate, with no obvious distress. Officers told crew that Christina and some friends at school frequently participate in cutting themselves. This evening Christina was angry at her mother so she cut herself, but the cut was too deep and this scared her, so she called 9-1-1. Patient confirmed this information. Patient cut her left wrist. Assessment of her wrists revealed several horizontal incisions. The cuts to her left wrist appeared to need sutures. Officer informed crew that patient's mother had been called and would meet the crew and her daughter at the hospital. Officer told crew that patient was under mental hygiene arrest due to intentional injury. Christina stated a razor blade was used to injure herself. Patient was cleared for any potential weapons by police officers. Patient escorted to the ambulance and secured to the gurney with the seat belts and shoulder harness. Officers followed crew to St. Mary's Hospital. En route to St. Mary's, patient was quiet, but cooperative. Patient remained alert and oriented during transport. On arrival at St. Mary's Hospital, patient was triaged and moved to the pediatric trauma bay and left in the care of Dr. Clasgens, the attending physician. **End of report**

CASE STUDY 14

Gynecologic Emergencies

Woman With Abdominal Pain

After completing a check of the ambulance, you receive a call to 2245 Twin Oakes Drive for an 18-year-old woman with abdominal pain and excessive vaginal bleeding. Time out is 1545.

Question 1

What are some of the possible causes of abdominal pain and excessive vaginal bleeding in an adolescent female?

A woman who appears to be in her late 40s greets you at the door and shows you into the single-family residence. She tells you that her daughter, Katrina, is upstairs in the bathroom. As you proceed up to the second-floor bathroom, the woman, Mrs. Whitman, tells you that Katrina has had nonstop vaginal bleeding for nearly 10 days. Today the bleeding got worse and was accompanied by cramps in her stomach.

"Katrina, dear, the ambulance people are here. May we come in?" Mrs. Whitman asks after knocking on the bathroom door.

"Yeah, come on in, Mom," Katrina replies.

When you open the door you are a bit surprised by what you see. A slightly obese adolescent is sitting in a bathtub full of red-stained water, which you presume is from blood. She has a large bath towel wrapped around her shoulders. After you introduce yourself, you ask, "What is going on today, Katrina?" She tells you that she was going through so many pads that she could not get dressed, so she opted for a bath instead. Now she is too weak to get out on her own. You complete a primary assessment **Table 1**.

Table 1	Primary Assessment Findings for Katrina
General impression	18-year-old woman reporting abdominal cramps and excessive vaginal bleeding.
Chief complaint	Excessive bleeding and abdominal cramping.
Mechanism of injury/nature of illness	No trauma. Appears to be gynecologic in nature.
Level of consciousness	Alert and oriented to person, place, time, and event.
Airway	Patent.
Breathing	Breathing is unlabored. Chest expansion is equal bilaterally. No trauma noted to the chest. Lung sounds are clear.
Circulation	Pulses present in both upper extremities. Skin is pale, moist, and warm. No bleeding from trauma, but vaginal bleeding is present.
Life threats	Excessive vaginal bleeding. Painful urination. Abdominal cramping.
Pertinent negatives	No trauma. No complaints of difficulty breathing. No shortness of breath. No loss of consciousness.
Pain	7 on a scale of 1 to 10.
Interventions	Sanitary pad to be placed at vaginal opening once out of the tub. High-flow oxygen administered via nonrebreathing mask due to excessive bleeding. Further assessment, treatment, and transport needed.

Due to the amount of blood loss, you request advanced life support (ALS). Your partner, Brianna, tells you that there are no paramedics currently available. You assess the patient's vital signs while she is in the water **Table 2** and ask Brianna to get the stair chair ready for transport out of the house and to the stretcher.

Table 2	Baseline Vital Signs for Katrina
Respirations	16 breaths/min and regular
Pulse	100 beats/min and regular
Skin	Warm, pale, and moist
Blood pressure	108/72 mm Hg
Oxygen saturation	98% on room air

You advise Katrina that she should be evaluated further at the hospital and that you are concerned about the amount of blood loss. Katrina agrees and asks her mother to retrieve her bathrobe and slippers. You and Brianna assist the patient to a standing position in the tub, while Katrina's mother helps to quickly dry her off with a towel. From there you assist Katrina out of the tub and onto the awaiting stair chair. Since ALS is not available, you opt to go to the closest hospital with your patient. You cover Katrina with some blankets from the ambulance and obtain a SAMPLE history from her including signs and symptoms, allergies, medications, pertinent past medical history, last oral intake, and events leading up to the illness or injury Table 3.

Table 3	SAMPLE History for Katrina
Signs and symptoms	Obvious vaginal bleeding.
	Patient reporting abdominal pain, painful urination, and abdominal bloating.
Allergies	No known drug allergies.
Medications	Birth control pills.
	Daily multivitamins.
Pertinent past medical history	Irregular periods 2 years ago.
	No other significant medical history.
Last oral intake	Breakfast at about 0930.
	Some fluids throughout the day (water and fruit juice).
Events leading up to the injury or illness	Period started 10 days ago. Got worse over the weekend with heavier flow this morning and the addition of intense abdominal pain and painful urination.

After obtaining the SAMPLE history you and your partner carry Katrina to the stretcher and then move her to the ambulance, where you continue your history taking Table 4.

Question 2

In addition to your SAMPLE history, what specific history questions should you ask of this patient on the basis of her signs and symptoms?

Question 3

Do you think it would be appropriate to have her mother present for the history taking? Why or why not?

Table 4 Additional History for Katrina

Pain	7 on a scale of 1 to 10.
Could you be pregnant?	No.
Have you ever been pregnant?	No.
How long have you been on birth control?	About 2 years.
How old were you when you first started menstruating?	14.
Are your periods usually regular?	They were irregular 2 years ago for a few months and no one knew why. They have been regular for 2 years up until this past month.
Are you sexually active?	No.
Why are you on birth control?	To control cycle regularity.
Do you smoke?	Yes, occasionally.
Have you ever had a sexually transmitted disease?	No.
Have you had any pelvic surgeries?	No.
Did you lose consciousness today?	No.

Katrina's mother tells you that she will meet you at Mercy Medical Center. Fortunately, Mercy Medical is only about a 15-minute drive from your current location.

Question 4

In which position would you transport Katrina? Why?

En route to the hospital you perform a secondary assessment **Table 5**.

Gynecologic Emergencies

Table 5 — Secondary Assessment Findings for Katrina

Level of consciousness	Alert and oriented to person, place, day, and event.
Airway	Patent.
Breathing	Rate is within normal limits.
	Lung sounds are clear and equal bilaterally.
	Oxygen is applied via nonrebreathing mask due to excessive blood loss.
Circulation	Pulses present in both upper extremities.
	Skin is pale, moist, and warm.
	No bleeding from trauma, but vaginal bleeding continues.
Head/neck	Trauma has been ruled out.
	No deformities, contusions, abrasions, punctures, penetrations, paradoxical motion in the chest, burns, tenderness, lacerations, or swelling (DCAP-BTLS) noted on head or neck.
Chest	No DCAP-BTLS noted to chest.
	Lung sounds are clear and equal bilaterally with full expansion.
Abdomen	Swollen, tender to the touch and painful.
	No rigidity, pulsating masses, or external bleeding noted.
	No DCAP-BTLS noted to abdomen.
Pelvis/genitalia	Pelvis is intact, no deformities or pain on palpation.
	Vaginal bleeding is heavy and continues en route to hospital.
Lower extremities	No DCAP-BTLS or pain noted.
	Pulse, movement, and sensation in lower extremities is present.
Upper extremities	No DCAP-BTLS or pain noted.
	Pulse, movement, and sensation in upper extremities is present.
Back/neck	No DCAP-BTLS noted.
Pain	Remains 7 out of 10.
Glasgow coma scale (GCS)	Score: 15 (eye opening, 4; verbal response, 5; motor response, 6).

Because of the patient's excessive vaginal bleeding, you ask Brianna to get another sanitary pad from the cabinet and secure it in place. In the 15 minutes during transport that your patient has been in the ambulance, she has already soaked two sanitary napkins. The used sanitary pads are saved in a red bag to take into triage.

Question 5

Why are the soaked pads important to give to the emergency department staff?

As Brianna calls ahead to the hospital, you obtain another set of vital signs on Katrina **Table 6**.

Table 6	Second Set of Vital Signs for Katrina
Respirations	20 breaths/min and regular
Pulse	112 beats/min and regular
Skin	Cool, pale, and moist
Blood pressure	106/70 mm Hg
Oxygen saturation	99% on oxygen

You note that Katrina's GCS score has now decreased to 14. You arrive at the hospital 16 minutes after leaving the residence. After giving a report to the triage nurse at the hospital, you are directed to bed 35L. You ask Katrina's mother to wait outside the room until you have her daughter settled in bed and pull the curtain for privacy. Dr. Murray enters the room along with a registered nurse, Heather. You hand off the red bag with soaked sanitary pads to the receiving staff. Dr. Murray has no further questions for you; therefore, you and Brianna wish Katrina well and head back to the ambulance.

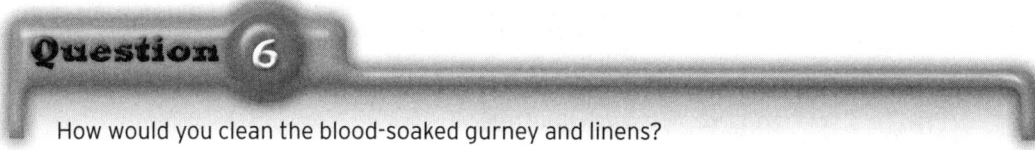

How would you clean the blood-soaked gurney and linens?

Case Analysis

It is estimated that approximately 1.4 million women visit emergency departments annually in the United States because of gynecologic emergencies. Pelvic pain, excessive vaginal bleeding, and pelvic infection are among the top three causes for these visits. When you assess female patients with abdominal discomfort and/or bleeding, gynecologic emergencies must not be ruled out. About 40% of women presenting with pelvic inflammatory disease are between the ages of 15 and 24 years. Any excessive or prolonged vaginal bleeding that occurs at the regular time of the menstrual cycle is known as menorrhagia.

■ Question 1

What are some of the possible causes of abdominal pain and excessive vaginal bleeding in an adolescent female?

The following are all possible causes of abdominal pain and excessive vaginal bleeding:
- Pregnancy
- Ectopic pregnancy
- Cancer of the uterus, vagina, cervix, and ovaries
- Certain drugs, especially anticoagulant drugs

- Inherited bleeding disorders such as von Willebrand's disease and hemophilia
- Trauma
- Premature menopause
- Uterine inflammation
- History of anticoagulant consumption
- Pelvic inflammatory disease

■ Question 2

What specific history questions should you ask of this patient on the basis of her signs and symptoms?

It is important to get a detailed history for this patient to help rule out certain causes. In addition to obtaining the SAMPLE history, be sure to ask the following questions:
- What is the mechanism of injury/nature of your illness?
- Could you be pregnant?
- Have you ever been pregnant?
- How old were you when you first started your periods?
- Are your periods usually regular?
- Are you sexually active?
- Are you taking birth control pills? If the answer to this question is "yes," also ask:
  - How long have you been on birth control?
  - Why are you on birth control?
- Do you smoke?
- Have you ever had a sexually transmitted disease?
- Have you had any pelvic surgeries?
- Did you lose consciousness today?
- Are you on any blood thinners?
- Do you have a bleeding disorder?

■ Question 3

Do you think it would be appropriate to have her mother present for the history taking? Why or why not?

In many states, the age of majority is 18 years. With that being the case, there is no legal obligation to have the mother (or any parent) present during the patient's assessment. This patient is entitled to her privacy if she so chooses. With any adolescent patient, however, it is important to consider her privacy when assessing and asking questions. Some teenagers may not be as willing to give honest answers to personal questions (such as, "Are you sexually active?") with parents present. Always keep the patient's best medical interest in mind. Check your state laws to determine what the age of majority is in your area. There are several professional techniques to gently remove a parent from a situation when you want to ask personal history questions. One way would be to have your partner distract the parent by asking her to come out into the hallway to give you demographic information. This way the parent still feels involved, but is not within hearing distance of the questions and answers.

Question 4

In which position would you transport Katrina? Why?

Most patients experiencing abdominal pain and discomfort are generally best transported with the legs flexed at the hips to relieve pressure from the abdomen. Because this patient has had significant blood loss, it is suggested that her head be lowered to increase blood flow to the heart and other vital organs. This position is called the shock position or Trendelenburg position. Katrina's legs could be flexed at the hips as well because you have ruled out any trauma.

Question 5

Why are the soaked pads important to give to the emergency department staff?

The soaked pads are evidence of the amount of blood loss. In addition to the soaked pads you can bring with you to the hospital, you will need to describe the amount of blood you saw at the scene (in the bathtub, for example). This information indicates the severity of the patient's condition.

Question 6

How would you clean the blood-soaked gurney and linens?

Clean-up procedures should follow your exposure control plan. This typically will involve cleaning the gurney and hard surfaces with a bleach solution. When you are done cleaning, all contaminated items should be disposed of in a red Occupational Safety and Health Administration (OSHA)–approved biohazard bag and discarded properly. All cleaning must be done while wearing personal protective equipment (PPE). At a minimum, gloves need to be worn. Depending on the amount of blood loss and the degree of potentially infectious substances, a gown and shoe coverings or booties may be appropriate. If the linens are cloth (versus disposable) they should be placed in a red OSHA-approved biohazard bag (separate from the disposable items) and properly washed.

Patient Care Report for Katrina

EMS Patient Care Report (PCR)

Date: 06-27-10	Incident No.: 201212	Nature of Call: Abdominal pain and bleeding		Location: 2245 Twin Oakes Drive	
Dispatched: 1543	En Route: 1545	At Scene: 1556	Transport: 1616	At Hospital: 1632	In Service: 1648

Patient Information

Age: 18 years	Allergies: No known drug allergies
Sex: Female	Medications: Ethinyl estradiol and norgestrel (Cryselle), multivitamins
Weight (in kg [lb]): 72.5 kg (160 lb)	Past Medical History: Irregular menstruation
	Chief Complaint: Excessive bleeding and abdominal pain

Vital Signs

Time	BP	Pulse	Respirations	SpO$_2$
1600	108/72	100 and regular	16 and regular	98% on room air
1610	106/70	112 and regular	20 and regular	99% on oxygen

EMS Treatment (circle all that apply)

Oxygen @ 15 L/min via (circle one): NC **(NRM)** Bag-Mask Device	Assisted Ventilation	Airway Adjunct	CPR
Defibrillation	**(Bleeding Control)**	Bandaging	Splinting	Other:

Narrative

Dispatched to a call for a woman experiencing abdominal pain and excessive vaginal bleeding. On arrival greeted at door by patient's mother and escorted to the upstairs bathroom, where the patient was found seated upright, unclothed, in the bathtub. Patient was alert and oriented to person, place, day/time, and event. The bathtub was full of reddish-tinged colored water. Patient stated she began her period 10 days ago but the bleeding got worse over the weekend. Patient described the bleeding as increasing in flow intensity accompanied by abdominal pain and cramping. Patient indicated she had a history of irregular periods about 2 years ago with no known etiology. Her menstrual cycle has been normal for the past 2 years until this past month. Patient denied being sexually active, denied ever being pregnant, denied having had any pelvic surgeries, and denied losing consciousness today or anytime leading up to this event. Patient admitted to smoking occasionally and is on birth control pills to help regulate her cycle. Patient denied any difficulty breathing. Patient last ate at approximately 0930 hours today. Patient believed she soaked through about 7–10 pads since this morning. Patient described her abdominal pain as cramping, and pain was rated as 7/10. Primary assessment findings are: patient has a patent airway and breathing is unlabored. Oxygen administered due to blood loss. Lung sounds were clear and equal bilaterally. Patient's skin is warm, pale, and moist while in the tub. Patient is not bleeding from any location other than the vagina. Pulses present in both upper extremities. Patient was assisted out of the tub by crew members and placed on the stair chair with a towel, a sanitary pad placed at the vaginal opening, and a bathrobe, slippers, and blankets. Patient placed on high-flow oxygen via nonrebreathing mask. Secondary assessment revealed the following: patient remained alert and oriented en route to hospital, airway remained patent, breathing was within normal range, lung sounds were clear and equal bilaterally. Oxygen remained in place for duration of transport. Pulses present in all four extremities; distal pulses weak and regular in rate. Skin was pale, warm, and moist. No trauma or DCAP-BTLS noted to any part of the body. Abdomen was swollen and tender to the touch; pain was a 7/10. GCS score was 15 at this time. Abdomen negative for pulsating masses and rigidity. Pelvis was intact; no deformities noted. Vaginal bleeding continued en route to hospital. Pulse, movement, and sensation were positive in all four extremities. GCS score decreased to a 14 during transport. BLS crew called for ALS but ALS not available, so patient transported to the nearest hospital. Patient left in the care of Dr. Murray and RN Heather. Bed rails placed in up position, bed lowered. Blankets left on patient. **End of report**

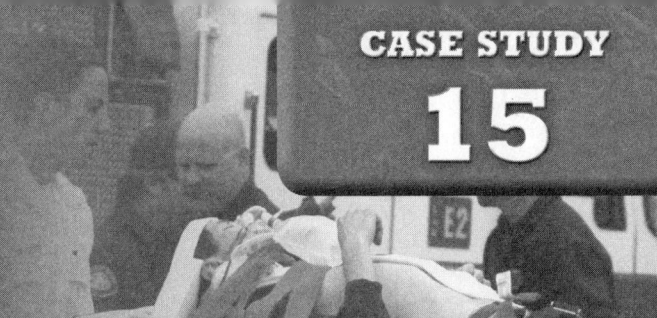

CASE STUDY 15

Bleeding

Man With a Forearm Laceration

While responding to a call for a 43-year-old man with a cut arm, you talk to your trainee, Rick, about what to possibly expect. Rick hopes to be licensed soon as an EMT and is under your supervision until he performs the required amount of patient care. He is a quick learner who is eager to obtain his EMT license.

Question 1

What advice do you have for your trainee partner on how to handle this call?

At 1815 hours you arrive at a single-family residence at 248 Barclay Square Drive to find a woman outside flagging you in. You enter through the garage, where you can see broken glass on the floor from a storm door that leads into the house. As you sidestep the broken glass, the woman introduces herself as Janet. She tells you that she was fighting with her husband, John, when he became angry and punched his hand through the window, cutting his forearm. You notice that you are following a trail of blood leading into the kitchen where John is sitting at the table. There is a blood-soaked towel haphazardly wrapped around his right forearm.

John looks up at you and says, "Hi … Boy, do I feel stupid."

John has a patent airway, is speaking in full sentences, and does not appear to be in any respiratory distress. He is shirtless and you quickly assess that there is no trauma to his head, neck, or chest. He also denies loss of consciousness or further injuries.

While you unwrap the towel and take a look at the wound, Rick grabs an 8″ × 10″ sterile trauma dressing from his kit to control the bleeding. John's eyes get big for a moment when he looks down at his wound. There is a 4″ (10 cm) laceration to his right forearm that needs suturing. While Rick is attempting to control the patient's bleeding, you gather the following information in a primary assessment Table 1 .

Bleeding

Table 1 — Primary Assessment Findings for John

General impression	43-year-old man with a cut on the right forearm with bleeding.
Chief complaint	Excessive bleeding on the right forearm and pain.
Mechanism of injury/nature of illness	Laceration on right forearm from glass.
Level of consciousness	Alert and oriented to person, place, time, and event.
Airway	Patent.
Breathing	Breathing is unlabored. Chest expansion is equal bilaterally. No trauma noted to the chest. Lung sounds are clear.
Circulation	Pulses are present in both upper extremities. Skin is pink, warm, and dry.
Life threats	Bleeding from the right forearm.
Pertinent negatives	No loss of consciousness. No fall or head trauma. No shortness of breath or chest pain. No dizziness or light-headedness.
Pain	Not assessed during primary assessment due to treatment of excessive bleeding.
Interventions	Direct pressure applied to control bleeding. High-flow oxygen administered via non-rebreathing mask due to excessive bleeding.

Question 2

What are your immediate priorities for this patient?

At this time, you notice that the wound is full thickness and that there is an additional blood-soaked towel on the kitchen table. You instruct Rick to grab another trauma dressing and apply immediate pressure to the wound.

With pressure being applied to the wound with a pressure dressing, Rick continues to ask the patient how he is feeling in order to ascertain changes in his level of consciousness. Meanwhile, you obtain a SAMPLE history from John, including signs and symptoms, allergies, medications, pertinent medical history, last oral intake, and the events leading up to the injury or illness Table 2.

Table 2	SAMPLE History for John
Signs and symptoms	Laceration to the right forearm. Pain at injury site. Uncontrolled bleeding.
Allergies	No known drug allergies.
Medications	Sertraline (Zoloft) Fenofibrate (Tricor)
Pertinent past medical history	History of depression. Recently diagnosed with high cholesterol.
Last oral intake	One light beer at about 1700 and a meatball sub at lunchtime.
Events leading up to the injury or illness	Argument with wife led to punching the window of the back storm door in the garage.

You inform the patient that the wound will require stitches. He asks to be taken to Rochester General Hospital, where his physician works. You tell John you want to transport him and begin to load him into the stair chair but he adamantly declines the offer and wants to walk to the ambulance.

Question 3

Would you allow a patient with severe bleeding to walk to the gurney? Why or why not?

You discuss your reason for using the stair chair with John and his wife. You explain that because of the amount of blood loss there is a risk for dizziness and loss of consciousness leading to further trauma. John then agrees and takes a seat on the stair chair.

Once inside the back of the ambulance, you notice that the patient's trauma dressings are soaked through with blood.

Question 4

How would you proceed with treatment of this patient?

Rick wants to add more bulky dressings on top of those already in place to stop the bleeding. You advise him, however, that a tourniquet will now be needed since the bleeding has not been controlled by direct pressure, elevation, and a pressure dressing. After you assist Rick in the application of a tourniquet above the level of bleeding, you then assess the patient's vital signs Table 3.

Table 3	Baseline Vital Signs for John
Respirations	16 breaths/min and regular
Pulse	110 beats/min and regular
Skin	Warm, pale, and moist
Blood pressure	134/88 mm Hg
Oxygen saturation	99% on oxygen

Due to the amount of bleeding John has experienced, you ask your driver to call for advanced life support (ALS) assistance en route. Your patient may need intravenous (IV) replacement fluids and possibly pain medication. Since Rochester General Hospital is 20 minutes from where you are, you decide it would be best to take him to the nearest emergency department, which is at Lakeside Memorial Hospital. ALS is on the way and will meet you off of an upcoming exit.

Question 5

While your partner is working on controlling the bleeding, what else could you do before meeting with ALS?

While en route, you complete a secondary assessment **Table 4**.

Table 4 — Secondary Assessment Findings for John

Level of consciousness	Alert and oriented to person, place, day, and event.
Airway	Patent.
Breathing	Rate is within normal limits.
	Lung sounds are clear and equal bilaterally.
	No trauma is noted to the chest.
	High-flow oxygen is applied via a nonrebreathing mask due to excessive blood loss.
Circulation	Pulses are present in the left upper extremity and absent in the right upper extremity due to application of a tourniquet.
	Skin is pale, moist, and warm.
Head/neck	Trauma has been ruled out.
	No deformities, contusions, abrasions, punctures, penetrations, paradoxical motion in the chest, burns, tenderness, lacerations, or swelling (DCAP-BTLS) are noted on head or the neck.
	Pupils are equal and reactive to light at 4 mm.
Chest	No DCAP-BTLS is noted to chest.
	Lung sounds are clear and equal bilaterally with full expansion.
Abdomen	Nontender, no distention or pain noted.
Pelvis/genitalia	Pelvis is intact, no deformities or pain on palpation.
Lower extremities	No DCAP-BTLS or pain noted.
	Pulse, movement, and sensation in lower extremities are present.
Upper extremities	No DCAP-BTLS or pain noted in left upper extremity.
	Pulse, movement, and sensation in left upper extremity are present.
Back/neck	No DCAP-BTLS noted.
Pain	6 on a scale of 1 to 10.
Glasgow coma scale (GCS)	Score: 15 (eye opening, 4; verbal response, 5; motor response, 6).

ALS is now on board and an IV line with pain medication is started. You obtain another set of vital signs **Table 5**.

Table 5 Second Set of Vital Signs for John

Respirations	14 breaths/min and regular
Pulse	100 beats/min and regular
Temperature	Warm, pale, and moist
Blood pressure	126/80 mm Hg
Oxygen saturation	99% on oxygen

Rick calls ahead to the emergency department staff to give them an update on John's condition. When you arrive, you bypass triage and head directly into the first trauma bay where the attending physician is waiting for you. After you relay your patient's medical information to the trauma team, the physician unwraps the bulky dressings to inspect the wound and blood spurts out several inches into the air. "Wow, John. You have a deep cut here. This is going to need more than stitches," the physician says. He tells his staff to call the operating room stat.

You wish John well and wash your hands before heading back to the ambulance.

Question 6

What appropriate measures should you now take to clean up the ambulance and yourself?

Case Analysis

Question 1

What advice do you have for your trainee partner on how to handle this call?

1. First and foremost, use standard precautions to protect yourself from any possible body fluids. If the dispatch information is correct and there is bleeding, gloves and eye protection must be worn, and a gown and mask must also be worn if you determine there is a risk of blood splatter.
2. Remain calm and professional, regardless of the situation. Do not let your adrenaline get the best of you during a trauma call.
3. Review the steps for bleeding control. First apply pressure over the wound using a dry, sterile dressing. Elevate the injury above the level of the heart if no fracture is suspected. If bleeding continues, apply a pressure dressing on top of the first dressing. If direct pressure with a dressing does not control the bleeding, apply a tourniquet above the level of bleeding.

Question 2

What are your immediate priorities for this patient?

With John's airway and breathing intact, your next immediate priority would be to stop the bleeding. You will need to place sterile trauma dressings and apply pressure to the wound. Even though this patient's quality of breathing is within normal limits (WNL), after bleeding is controlled, provide high-flow oxygen to the patient due to the severity and amount of bleeding.

■ Question 3

Would you allow a patient with severe bleeding to walk to the gurney? Why or why not?

This patient should not be allowed to walk to the gurney because of the amount of blood loss. A sudden change in elevation (standing up, for example) could cause this patient to faint, resulting in further trauma.

■ Question 4

How would you proceed with treatment of this patient?

If the direct pressure and pressure bandages do not stop the bleeding, consider the use of a tourniquet. Many commercial tourniquets are now available, but if you do not have access to a commercial tourniquet, you can make your own out of cravats, for example, or a blood pressure cuff. The tourniquet should be placed above the level of the bleeding. Once the tourniquet is applied, it should stay in place until arrival at the hospital and evaluation by a physician or until medical control or local protocols indicate you may remove it. Be sure to mark the time of placement on the tourniquet and notify the health care facility that a tourniquet has been applied. If you do use a blood pressure cuff as a tourniquet, be certain to tell the emergency department staff so they do not remove the cuff hastily.

■ Question 5

While your partner is working on controlling the bleeding, what else could you do before meeting with ALS?

Treat the patient for shock. Administer high-flow oxygen, and keep the patient warm and calm. Reassess the patient's airway, breathing, and circulation and assess your interventions. Call ahead to the emergency department so the staff knows what to expect upon your arrival. It is possible that your patient will need surgery to repair an artery to stop the bleeding.

■ Question 6

What appropriate measures should you now take to clean up the ambulance and yourself?

Cleanup procedures should follow your exposure control plan. This typically will involve cleaning the gurney and hard surfaces with a bleach solution. When you are done with the paper towels, they should be bagged and tagged in a red biohazard bag and disposed of properly. All cleaning must be done while you are wearing personal protective equipment (PPE). At a minimum, you and your crew should wear gloves and eye protection. Depending on the amount of blood loss and the degree of mess, a gown and shoe coverings or booties may be appropriate. Your exposure control plan should also indicate what to do if your uniform has become exposed to blood or other body fluids. Agencies are required to have laundry facilities for exposed clothing and linens separate from laundry facilities that are used for the base or station, such as bed linens for the crews.

Patient Care Report for John

EMS Patient Care Report (PCR)

Date: 05-21-2012	Incident No.: 12755	Nature of Call: Laceration to the arm	Location: 248 Barclay Square Drive	
Dispatched: 1802	En Route: 1804	At Scene: 1815	Transport: 1826	At Hospital: 1839	In Service: 1904

Patient Information

Age: 43	**Allergies:** No known drug allergies
Sex: Male	**Medications:** Sertraline (Zoloft), fenofibrate (Tricor)
Weight (in kg [lb]): 99 kg (220 lb)	**Past Medical History:** Depression, high cholesterol
	Chief Complaint: Laceration to right forearm and pain

Vital Signs

Time	BP	Pulse	Respirations	SpO$_2$
1825	134/88	110 and regular	16 and regular	99% on oxygen
1830	126/80	100 and regular	14 and regular	99% on oxygen

EMS Treatment (circle all that apply)

Oxygen @ **15** L/min via (circle one): NC **(NRM)** Bag-mask device	Assisted Ventilation	Airway Adjunct	CPR
Defibrillation	**(Bleeding Control)**	**(Bandaging)**	Splinting	Other:

Narrative

Dispatched to the home of a 43-year-old man with a laceration to the forearm from punching the glass window of the back door in the garage. Greeted in driveway by patient's wife. Patient found seated in kitchen, alert and oriented with a patent airway. Blood-soaked towel was wrapped around injured forearm. Patient denied losing consciousness, feeling dizzy, light-headed, or falling. Patient also denied having any chest pain or difficulty breathing. Primary assessment revealed a patent airway, unlabored breathing with equal chest expansion, and no trauma to the chest. Pulses were present in both upper extremities, and skin was pink, warm, and moist. Vital signs as noted above. Bleeding noted to right forearm bandaged with sterile dressing. Patient placed on high-flow oxygen via nonrebreathing mask. Patient moved to ambulance via stair chair and gurney for transport to Lakeside Memorial Hospital. Met ALS paramedic Terry. Secondary assessment findings revealed the patient was alert and oriented, airway was patent, lung sounds were clear, and chest expansion remained equal bilaterally. Pulses were present in both extremities, and skin was pale, moist, and warm. Trauma to the head and neck were ruled out; pupils were equal and reactive to light; abdomen was nontender with no distention or pain; pelvis was intact, with no deformities or pain; no DCAP-BTLS noted to the lower extremities; pulse, movement, and sensation were positive in lower extremities; no DCAP-BTLS noted to the back; pain was rated as 6/10; and GCS score was 15. Patient was transferred directly to awaiting emergency department staff in the trauma bay without incident. **End of report**

CASE STUDY 16

Soft-Tissue Injuries

Girl With Dog Bites

Shortly after completing the ambulance check for your afternoon shift, the tones sound for your first call of the day. The dispatcher informs you that an 8-year-old girl has been bitten by a dog. Dispatch also tells you that the girl is conscious and alert at this time. You are dispatched to 80 Reynolds Road at 1221 hours. En route to the call, you talk to your driver about the possible extent of injury to the girl and contact the dispatcher to inquire about the location of the dog.

Question 1

What should you consider during the scene size-up for this call?

On arrival, you are welcomed into the residence by a woman who identifies herself as a neighbor, and you find the girl, Delaney, sitting upright on the couch in the living room. The dog's owner is present; she tells you that the dog that bit Delaney is a 70-lb golden retriever and confirms that the dog is at her home. You can see that your patient has been crying.

Question 2

What approach would you use to calm and reassure this young patient?

Because the patient is talking in full sentences as you approach, you know that she has a patent airway. You also notice that she is tracking you and making an attempt to wipe her tear-stained cheeks and smile. Delaney says that she does not live at this address and that her father is on his way over. You see a puncture wound indicative of a dog bite on Delaney's left forearm, just above the wrist. You gently place your hand on Delaney's uninjured arm and notice that her skin is warm and dry and that she has a bounding radial pulse. The bleeding on the injured arm has been controlled and the wound does not appear to need sutures. You offer Delaney a small stuffed animal from your pediatric kit to hold before you proceed with the assessment **Table 1**. One of the adults tells you the girl was also bitten on the stomach.

Table 1 — Primary Assessment Findings for Delaney

General impression	8-year-old girl with a dog bite to her left arm.
Chief complaint	Pain at injury site.
Level of consciousness	Alert and oriented to person, place, time, and event.
Airway	Patent.
Breathing	Breathing is unlabored. Chest expansion is equal bilaterally. No trauma noted to the chest. Lung sounds are clear.
Circulation	Pulses present in both upper extremities. Skin is pink, warm, and dry. Bleeding at the arm has been controlled. There is a small open wound on the stomach, but it is not bleeding.
Life threats	No life threats at this time.
Pertinent negatives	Patient has no difficulty breathing. Patient reports no pain other than at wound sites. Patient denies loss of consciousness.
Interventions	Comfort care, bandage wound site.
Pain	The patient is unable to articulate a number on the pain scale at this time.

Question 3

Should you begin treatment of this patient before the girl's father is present?

Question 4

What concerns might you have about the dog that bit this patient?

Question 5

How should you address and treat the wound to the patient's arm and stomach?

As you are finishing your primary assessment with Delaney, her father walks through the front door. He approaches Delaney calmly and asks to see her injuries. The owner of the dog is distraught over the dog bite and very apologetic to both Delaney and her father. She offers to show him proof of rabies vaccination and all other canine immunizations for her dog.

You bandage both wounds using sterile 4″ × 4″ pads and tape. You begin obtaining a SAMPLE history, including signs and symptoms, allergies, medications, pertinent medical history, last oral intake, and events leading up to the injury or illness **Table 2**.

Soft-Tissue Injuries

Table 2 SAMPLE History for Delaney

Signs and symptoms	Bite wound to the left forearm above the wrist and on the stomach
	Minimal bleeding to the arm, no bleeding to the stomach wound
	Pain to the bite areas
Allergies	No known drug allergies
	Allergies only to seasonal pollen
Medications	Diphenhydramine (Children's Benadryl), as needed
Pertinent medical history	No medical history other than the seasonal allergies
Last oral intake	Last ate at breakfast (scrambled eggs, toast, and milk) around 0930
Events leading up to the injury or illness	The child ran into the yard to retrieve a ball when the dog ran at her and bit her on the arm and stomach

Through questioning, you find that Delaney was running into the front yard of the neighbor's house to retrieve a ball. When she ran into the yard, the dog lunged at her and bit her on the arm and stomach. After having a firm grasp of the event, you ask Delaney and her father if it would be okay to assess her vital signs **Table 3**.

Table 3 Baseline Vital Signs for Delaney

Respirations	22 breaths/min and regular
Pulse	112 beats/min and regular
Skin	Pink, warm, and dry
Blood pressure	108/62 mm Hg
Oxygen saturation	99% on room air

As you finish your primary assessment and history taking, your driver gives you demographic information for Delaney, including the name of her pediatrician, Dr. Kaplan. You suggest transporting Delaney to Strong Memorial Hospital, but her father says he would rather take Delaney to Dr. Kaplan directly.

Question 6

Do you agree with the actions of the patient's father? Why or why not?

Question 7

What approach would you use to ensure that the patient's father is making an informed decision not to transport the patient to the hospital via ambulance?

Although you explain to the father that Delaney should be transported by ambulance to the hospital, he maintains his decision to take his daughter to see Dr. Kaplan. He agrees that she should be seen as soon as possible and assures you that he will contact the pediatrician immediately. You explain the potential consequences of not seeking treatment, and he understands the probability that follow-up antibiotics will be needed. He willingly signs the medical refusal form after reading over the refusal statement; his neighbor signs as a witness. You write down follow-up instructions for him as a professional reminder and let him know that you can return if he changes his mind. You make sure that you have documented your assessment findings, the emergency care that you provided, your efforts to obtain consent for transport and further treatment, and the responses to your efforts. You wish Delaney well, and depart from the scene to begin your documentation of this call and to review reporting requirements for dog bites in your jurisdiction. Time back in service is 1302 hours.

Question 8

What specific information would you want to be sure to include on the PCR for this patient (apart from demographics, traditional narrative information, and run times)?

Case Analysis

■ Question 1

What should you consider during the scene size-up for this call?

Scene safety is a priority. In this case you should be concerned with the location of the dog. Is the dog still on the loose? Where is the dog being held? Is there more than one dog? Are there adults on scene or only a child? En route to the call, contact dispatch to ask whether the dog has been secured, if you have not already been given that information.

■ Question 2

What approach would you use to calm and reassure this young patient?

As with any patient, maintaining a professional, calm demeanor is the first step in approaching patients. When you are caring for children, it is especially important to remain calm and friendly. Children can often pick up on and react to the feelings of adults and others around them. A calm adult helps to contribute to a calm child. Kneeling down to approach the patient at her level is one way to help gain the patient's trust.

■ Question 3

Should you begin treatment of this patient before the girl's father is present?

Although this patient is a minor and parental consent is preferred, you should always act in the best medical interest of the patient. In a situation like this you may use implied consent to treat a minor whose parent is not available to grant permission. Implied consent in this scenario would assume that the parents and/or guardians would consent to care if they were there to do so.

■ Question 4

Now that you have confirmed your patient has been bitten by a dog on the arm and the stomach, what concerns might you have about the dog that bit her?

Several concerns come to mind with an injury involving a dog bite, including the following:
- Is the dog a stray?
- Where is the dog?
- Is the dog in the area of the EMS providers?
- Has the dog bitten anyone else recently?
- Are there any other hidden dog bites on the patient?
- Could the dog possibly have rabies?
- If the dog has an owner, does the dog have a vaccination history, and, if so, could you have access to the vaccination records?

You will also need to know the reporting procedures in your state for dog bites. Some states and counties require that all dog bites be reported. A number of states require that dog bites be reported to local health departments, whereas others want dog bites reported to animal control. Check with your state or regional authorities on the laws specific to your response area.

■ Question 5

How should you address and treat the wound to the patient's arm?

A dog bite wound should be treated similarly to any other type of open wound to an extremity. Standard precautions, such as personal protective equipment (PPE) for providers, are necessary. Keep in mind that infection is always a possibility with any open wound, so sterile dressings should be used whenever available.

Question 6

Do you agree with the actions of the patient's father? Why or why not?

Delaney's father has the right to seek treatment through the family's personal pediatrician. Because her vital signs are stable and she has no compromise to her airway, breathing, or circulation, it is acceptable to allow the patient's father to sign a release for her. If the father made no mention of seeking further treatment for this child and the wound needed sutures, an argument could then be made that the child should be transported to the local emergency department.

Question 7

What approach would you use to ensure that the patient's father is making an informed decision not to transport the patient to the hospital via ambulance?

Discussing your assessment findings as well as the need for immediate further care to the patient's father is one way to ensure an informed decision is being made. Making certain that parents understand any potential complications from refusal of care is key to informed consent. Have parents repeat back to you their understanding of the situation. Also encourage them to call for another ambulance at any time if they change their minds.

Question 8

What specific information would you want to be sure to include on the PCR for this patient (apart from demographics, traditional narrative information, and run times)?

A call is never finished until thorough documentation is completed. Apart from your assessment findings and treatment, be sure to include the following in this PCR:
- An indication that the child was found in the presence of unrelated adults
- A notation that the child's father did arrive at the scene
- Documentation that the child's father understood (was informed) about his decision to seek treatment through a personal physician versus being transported to the emergency department
- Notation that the dog was secured away from the scene
- Notation that you were able to review the dog's vaccination record (write down those vaccinations with which the dog is up-to-date)
- The size of the wounds and depth
- Whether this event was witnessed or not
- Any bystander comments relating to the call

Patient Care Report for Delaney

EMS Patient Care Report (PCR)

Date: 07-12-11	Incident No.: 011456	Nature of Call: Dog bite	Location: 80 Reynolds Road	
Dispatched: 1221	En Route: 1222	At Scene: 1230	Transport:	At Hospital:	In Service: 1302

Patient Information

Age: 8 years	**Allergies:** Seasonal only
Sex: Female	**Medications:** Diphenhydramine (Children's Benadryl) as needed
Weight (in kg [lb]): 30 kg/67 lb	**Past Medical History:** Seasonal allergies
	Chief Complaint: Dog bites to arm and stomach

Vital Signs

Time: 1236	BP: 108/62	Pulse: 112 and regular	Respirations: 22 and regular	Spo₂: 99% on room air
Time:	BP:	Pulse:	Respirations:	Spo₂:
Time:	BP:	Pulse:	Respirations:	Spo₂:

EMS Treatment
(circle all that apply)

Oxygen @ ____ L/min via (circle one): NC NRM Bag-mask Device	Assisted Ventilation	Airway Adjunct	CPR
Defibrillation	Bleeding Control	**(Bandaging)**	Splinting	Other:

Narrative

Dispatched to residence for an 8-year-old girl with dog bites. Dog secured at a separate location. On arrival on scene, patient found in the single-family residence with a neighbor, sitting on the couch in the living room. Patient made eye contact and appeared to have been crying. Patient had a patent airway and was alert and oriented. Breathing was unlabored and chest expansion was equal bilaterally. Skin was warm, pink, and dry, and the bleeding at the wound on her left arm had been controlled. Patient's parents were not present initially; however, patient's father showed up at approximately 1234 hours. On further assessment, a small puncture wound was found to the patient's stomach, just above the navel. This wound was not bleeding, but a puncture was noted. Both wounds were covered with sterile dressings and tape. Witnesses to the event denied loss of consciousness to the patient. Patient denied feeling dizzy or sick to her stomach. Patient's father was advised of the need for further wound care, but refused ambulance transport. Crew strongly recommended father to seek out Delaney's pediatrician for follow-up care and informed him of the possibility of infection at the wound site. Patient's father indicated that he would take Delaney to her pediatrician, Dr. Kaplan, later today. Patient's father and witness signed medical refusal form. **End of report**

Case Study 17

Face and Neck Injuries

Adolescent Softball Pitcher With a Facial Injury

It is a warm spring afternoon and you and your partner, Tim, are at the high school on EMS standby for a softball game. At the top of the third inning, a line drive is hit and you notice the pitcher collapses to the ground. The umpire calls a time out and the coaches run onto the field. The pitcher has been struck in the face by the line-drive ball. You run to her aid as Tim calls the incident in to the emergency medical services (EMS) dispatcher and requests advanced life support (ALS) to the scene. He grabs equipment from the ambulance and heads onto the field to assist you.

Question 1

On the basis of the mechanism of injury for this patient, what immediate equipment needs do you anticipate?

Question 2

What assessment approach would you take with this patient?

The players head off the field as you approach the patient. She is crying out in pain but tracking you as you walk up. You introduce yourself and she tells you that her name is Katherine. You ask the coach to manually stabilize her cervical spine while you remove her mouth guard and assess the extent of her injuries **Table 1**. The patient's airway is intact, although you notice that she is bleeding from the nose. Tim places her on blow-by oxygen with a nonrebreathing mask and you apply a cold pack to the nose.

Question 3

What are some of your immediate concerns for this patient?

Table 1 — Primary Assessment Findings for Katherine

General impression	16-year-old girl, hit in face by line-drive softball, lying in the pitcher's circle, conscious and crying.
Chief complaint	Severe pain to the nose and face.
	Headache.
Mechanism of injury/nature of illness	Struck in the face by softball line drive.
Level of consciousness	Alert and oriented to person, place, day, time, and event.
Airway	Intact, but bleeding from nose. Teeth are fully intact; patient was wearing a mouth guard.
Breathing	Breathing is shallow and equal bilaterally.
	No complaints of difficulty breathing.
	No deformities, contusions, abrasions, punctures, penetrations, paradoxical motion in the chest, burns, tenderness, lacerations, or swelling (DCAP-BTLS) noted to the chest.
	High-flow oxygen administered via nonrebreathing mask due to mechanism of injury and possible head injury.
Circulation	Pulses present in both upper extremities.
	Bleeding from the nose is noted at the apparent point of impact.
	Skin is warm, pale, and dry.
Life threats	Facial injury, possible neck and head injuries.
Pertinent negatives	No loss of consciousness but has neck pain and chest pain.
Pain	10 on a scale of 1 to 10.
Glasgow coma scale (GCS)	Score: 15 (eye opening, 4; verbal response, 5; motor response, 6).
Interventions	Cervical spine stabilization.
	Cold pack applied to the nose to control bleeding and swelling.
	Suction to nares to remove blood and secretions.
	Oxygen administration via nonrebreathing mask.

You obtain a set of vital signs from Katherine **Table 2**.

Table 2 — Baseline Vital Signs for Katherine

Respirations	26 breaths/min and shallow
Pulse	130 and regular
Skin	Warm, dry, and pale
Blood pressure	118/78 mm Hg
Oxygen saturation	100% on oxygen

Question 4

What can you do to both help alleviate pain at the impact site and control bleeding?

Katherine's parents have arrived at her side and are providing support for her. While you continue with your assessment, Katherine's mother holds the cold pack to her daughter's nose. You explain to them that you will need to immobilize Katherine on a backboard as a precaution before moving her to the ambulance. After applying a cervical collar, you log roll the patient and assess her back before securing her to the backboard. You move her to the back of the ambulance and obtain a SAMPLE history, including signs and symptoms, allergies, medications, pertinent past medical history, last oral intake, and events leading up to the injury or illness Table 3.

Table 3 SAMPLE History for Katherine

Signs and symptoms	Swelling and bleeding on the nose and face.
	Patient reporting pain to her nose and face as well as headache and nausea.
Allergies	Seafood and penicillin.
Medications	Daily vitamins plus iron and calcium.
	No prescribed medications.
Pertinent past medical history	No significant medical history other than an occasional ear infection.
Last oral intake	Lunch at approximately 3 hours prior to the game. Water drunk between innings.
Events leading up to the injury or illness	During a softball game, line-drive ball hit pitcher in the face.
	EMS crew witnessed the event.

Once in the back of the ambulance, Katherine remains calm but begins to cough because she is aspirating blood from the nasal injury. You immediately apply external suctioning and replace the blow-by oxygen. The cold pack has helped to relieve some of her pain, which she now rates as 8 out of 10. The closest trauma center is approximately 15 miles away, so you decide it would be best to rendezvous with ALS en route to the facility. After you reassess Katherine's airway and breathing, you perform a secondary assessment Table 4.

Table 4 — Secondary Assessment Findings for Katherine

Level of consciousness	Alert and oriented to person, place, day, and event.
Airway	Intact and patent, although suctioning is needed to keep airway clear of blood and other fluids.
Breathing	26 breaths/min and shallow with equal, bilateral chest rise and fall.
Circulation	Pulses present in both upper extremities, strong and regular.
	Skin is warm, pale, and dry.
Head/neck	Patient complaining of increased headache and pain to injury at the bridge of her nose.
	Bruising now noted to the injury site along with significant swelling.
	Nasal bleeding still present but controlled with suctioning and a cold pack.
	No other DCAP-BTLS noted on head or neck.
	No pain to the neck.
	Pupils are equal and reactive at 4 mm.
Chest	No DCAP-BTLS noted to the chest.
	Lung sounds are clear and equal bilaterally with full expansion.
Abdomen	Soft, nontender, no rigidity.
	Increased nausea reported.
Pelvis/genitalia	Intact pelvis, and no deformities or pain on palpation.
	No pain to genitalia; inspection is deferred.
Lower extremities	Pulse, movement, and sensation present in lower extremities.
	No injuries noted to lower extremities.
Upper extremities	Pulse, movement, and sensation present in upper extremities.
	No DCAP-BTLS noted to upper extremities.
Back/neck	Patient complaining of soreness to upper part of the back.
	No visible injury noted when inspected before immobilization.
Pain	Facial pain 8 out of 10.
	Headache pain 6 out of 10.
Glasgow coma scale (GCS)	Score: 15 (eye opening, 4; verbal response, 5; motor response, 6).

Just as you complete the secondary assessment on Katherine, Tim tells you that ALS is up ahead in the gas station parking lot.

Question 5

What potential changes in signs and symptoms should be of particular concern to you and why?

ALS is now on board and you continue with basic life support care. You reassess Katherine's airway and suction her nose once again. This time there is not nearly as much fluid to suction as before. You are relieved that the bleeding has slowed down considerably.

As the paramedic establishes an intravenous line, you call the trauma center staff to let them know your estimated time of arrival is about 10 minutes.

Question 6

What is the most important information to share with the triage nurse once you are in the emergency department?

After you arrive at the hospital and give the pediatric triage nurse the report, you and your crew move Katherine to the pediatric emergency department, trauma bed 2. You leave Katherine's belongings with her mother. You wish Katherine a speedy recovery and hope that she will be back on the field in the near future.

Case Analysis

Facial trauma (also known as maxillofacial injury) includes, in general, injury to the mouth, face, and jaw. Broken bones are common in facial trauma, but injury can affect soft tissue as well as the eyes. Nasal fractures are the most common type of broken bones to the face. Young children and infants with facial fractures need special treatment by maxillofacial surgeons because their bones are still growing. Considering the position of the pitcher, there is a high incidence of maxillofacial injuries in softball.

■ Question 1

On the basis of the mechanism of injury for this patient, what immediate equipment needs do you anticipate?

A fully stocked medic bag (with oxygen tank and oxygen delivery devices), cervical collars, a backboard, and a suction unit should be brought to the patient on this call.

■ Question 2

What assessment approach would you take with this patient?

Your assessment approach to this patient should be calm, professional, and in control. Due to the mechanism of injury, spinal stabilization is a priority followed by immediate airway management.

■ Question 3

What are some of your immediate concerns for this patient?

Airway and breathing would be immediate concerns for this patient. Since she was struck in the face, there is a great deal of potential for facial trauma, which could impact airway patency. Suction should be immediately available to clear the airway as needed. Head and neck trauma are also immediate concerns.

■ **Question 4**

What can you do to both help alleviate pain at the impact site and control bleeding?

Cold packs should be used to help alleviate pain and minimize bleeding. The cold will constrict the blood vessels and assist in bleeding control. Anytime cold packs are used, they must be wrapped first in cloth, such as a cravat, before applying to the wound site. Never place cold packs or ice directly onto skin as this could cause permanent tissue damage (frostbite).

■ **Question 5**

What potential changes in signs and symptoms should be of particular concern to you and why?

Changes to Katherine's level of consciousness would be of concern to you since this is often the first notable indication of traumatic brain injury. Changes in the GCS score are also significant. According to the Brain Trauma Foundation, a drop in the score to less than 9 or a decrease of more than 2 points at any time doubles the chance of death in that patient. Pupils should also be checked and rechecked. The cranial nerves in the brain that control the pupils are very sensitive to pressures in the brain. Uneven pupils often represent an increase in intracranial pressure. In addition, monitor the patient carefully for airway problems, including aspiration of blood and respiratory failure.

■ **Question 6**

What is the most important information to share with the triage nurse once you are in the emergency department?

Certainly sharing the mechanism of injury with the triage nurse is important. Also advise the staff that Katherine did not lose consciousness and that her level of consciousness did not change. Finally, be sure to advise the nurse that suctioning/cold packs were needed to manage the patient's airway.

Patient Care Report for Katherine

EMS Patient Care Report (PCR)

Date: 05-02-2011	Incident No.: 782	Nature of Call: Person struck in face with softball	Location: 1150 Winton Road South	
Dispatched:	En Route:	At Scene: 1645	Transport: 1655	At Hospital: 1715	In Service: 1750

Patient Information

Age: 16 years	Allergies: Seafood and penicillin
Sex: Female	Medications: Vitamins, iron, and calcium
Weight (in kg [lb]): 65 kg (145 lb)	Past Medical History: None
	Chief Complaint: Pain in the face

Vital Signs

Time	BP	Pulse	Respirations	SpO$_2$
1654	118/78	130 and regular	26 and shallow	100% on oxygen
1701	116/76	98 and regular	18 and regular	100% on oxygen

EMS Treatment (circle all that apply)

Oxygen @ <u>15</u> L/min via (circle one): NC **(NRM)** Bag-mask device	Assisted Ventilation	Airway Adjunct	CPR
Defibrillation	**(Bleeding Control)**	Bandaging	**(Splinting** Full Spinal Immobilization**)**	**(Other:)** Suction

Narrative

Crew witnessed a 16-year-old female softball pitcher struck in the face with a line drive. Patient collapsed to the ground but did not lose consciousness. Crew attended to patient immediately. ALS promptly requested to the scene. Patient was alert and oriented and crying out in pain. Manual head stabilization held by softball coach. Patient's airway was intact; however, she was bleeding from the nose. Oxygen was given via nonrebreathing mask and blow-by method while blood and secretions were suctioned from the nose. Cold pack applied to the bridge of the nose for pain and bleeding control. Mouth guard was worn at time of impact; teeth are fully intact. Mouth guard removed by crew and given to patient's parents for safe keeping. Breathing was shallow, but equal expansion was noted. No trauma to the chest or neck. Pulses were strong in both upper extremities; skin was warm, pale, and dry. Some bleeding was noted to the nose at point of impact. Patient's parents were on scene at the time of the injury. Initial GCS score was 15. Patient immobilized and moved to the back of the ambulance for history and secondary assessment. Secondary assessment revealed swelling and minor bleeding to the nose and face; patient complained of headache and facial pain; patient's oropharynx was suctioned due to blood dripping down back of nasopharynx. Cryotherapy continued en route to the hospital. Initial facial pain was 10/10; after we applied chemical cold pack for a few minutes, pain decreased to 8/10. Pulses present in all four extremities, skin was warm, pale, and dry. Patient then reported increasing headache and pain to injury at bridge of nose. Bruising noted to the injury site along with significant swelling to the face. Nasal bleeding was still present, but slowed and controlled with suctioning. Patient denied any neck pain. Pupils were equal and reactive to light at approximately 4 mm. No DCAP-BTLS noted to the chest. Abdomen was soft and nontender without rigidity. Patient reported feeling nauseous. Pelvis was intact with no deformities or pain noted. Patient denied pain to genitalia region; inspection deferred. Pulse, movement, and sensation were present in both lower and upper extremities; no injuries noted. En route, patient felt soreness to upper back. No visible injury noted prior to placing her on backboard. Pain remained 8/10. Headache pain was rated 6/10. On reassessment, GCS score was 15; no change. Paramedic rendezvoused en route to the hospital. Patient transferred to hospital staff, with parents present, without incident. **End of report**

CASE STUDY 18

Head and Spine Injuries

Possible Neck Injury in a Swimming Pool

It is 2330 hours and you and your partner, Alex, have just settled down in the bunk room for what you are hoping will be a quiet night. You are tired from a long day in the hot, humid weather and fall asleep rather quickly. Just as you drift off, the tones sound and you hear the dispatcher come across with a call. As you pry your eyes open and sit up, you cannot believe what you are hearing. The call is for a 21-year-old man in a swimming pool with a possible neck injury. Alex is already up and confirming the call with the dispatcher as you head out toward the ambulance. The call location is 1468 David Avenue, and your time out is 2334 hours. Dispatch further advises that due to the nature of the call, advanced life support (ALS) has also been dispatched.

Question 1

What are your scene size-up thoughts for this call?

You arrive at the call location at 2348 hours. As Alex pulls the ambulance up to the house, you see a few young adults waving you down from the front yard. The house is a single-family, two-story colonial residence. There are cars parked in the driveway, front yard, and on the street as well. As you are escorted around to the back of the house, you sense their concern. During the short walk, they are quickly explaining what happened.

They were having a pool party when their friend, Daniel, decided to do flips into the pool. As you enter the backyard, you see a 4' above-ground pool. You wonder to yourself how someone could be doing flips into an above-ground pool. The young woman who is walking you to the backyard explains that the patient had flipped off of the second-story balcony into the pool several times. She proceeds to tell you that on the last jump, Daniel hit the bottom of the pool and could no longer move. When Daniel's friends realized that he was not surfacing, they jumped in the water to help him. As you approach the side of the pool, you find your patient prone in the water. Four of his friends are each holding him up by a limb, just high enough out of the water so that he can breathe. He is crying out.

Question 2

What is the best way to remove this patient from the pool? What special considerations do you have for securing him to a backboard?

You introduce yourself to Daniel and ask him a few questions to ascertain his level of consciousness. He is painfully aware of his surroundings and what happened to him. He also knows what day it is. After you determine that Daniel is alert, you ask if he lost consciousness. He says he did not. His friends do not believe he lost consciousness either. You then ask Daniel if anything hurts. He yells out, "No, but I can't move my arms or legs!" You obtain a radial pulse and find it strong but slow. You do not note any bleeding. It is difficult to determine his skin color in the water and in this light. His skin is cool to the touch, but you are not surprised by this because Daniel has been in the water for approximately 20 minutes.

Your supervisor arrives on the scene to offer assistance. Since Daniel's friends are already in the water holding him up, you decide to have them assist in getting Daniel on the board. Alex comes back with the backboard, straps, head blocks, and cervical collar. You are close enough to reach Daniel's head for stabilization. You explain to Daniel and his friends your plan for moving him to the backboard. Alex moves the board into the water and positions the board near the patient. You take a position at the patient's head and place the cervical collar around his neck. Alex submerges the board and carefully brings it up next to the patient. On your count, the unit rolls Daniel into a supine position in the water onto the awaiting backboard. The patient is lifted out of the water on the backboard and placed on the gurney. You quickly cover him with blankets and attempt to dry him off as best you can. Now that Daniel is out of the water and in a supine position, you can take a better look at him and assess his breathing. You note that his face is pale but his chest is somewhat flushed. He is also having some difficulty breathing.

Question 3

What treatment should you initiate before moving him to the ambulance?

Alex hands you a nonrebreathing mask with the oxygen set at 15 L/min and you explain to Daniel that you are giving him some oxygen to help him breathe. After the oxygen is secure, you perform a primary assessment Table 1 .

Table 1 — Primary Assessment Findings for Daniel

General impression	21-year-old man found in swimming pool unable to move.
Chief complaint	Unable to move.
Mechanism of injury/nature of illness	Jump into pool, hitting neck on the bottom of pool.
Level of consciousness	Alert and oriented to person, place, time, and event.
Airway	Patent.
Breathing	Breathing is shallow. Chest expansion is equal bilaterally. No trauma noted to the chest. Lung sounds are clear.
Circulation	Pulses are strong but slow in the upper extremities. Skin is pale to the face, but flushed at the core, cool, and moist.
Life threats	Difficulty breathing and paralysis.
Pertinent negatives	Patient denies loss of consciousness.
Interventions	High-flow oxygen via nonrebreathing mask. Full spinal immobilization. Dried off and warmed.
Pain	None.

Once the patient is dried off, secured to the backboard, covered with blankets, and oxygen has been administered, he is moved toward the ambulance. Once you reach the back of the ambulance, you gather a SAMPLE history, including signs and symptoms, allergies, medications, pertinent past medical history, last oral intake, and events leading up to the injury or illness **Table 2**.

Table 2 — SAMPLE History for Daniel

Signs and symptoms	Paralysis, difficulty breathing.
Allergies	No known drug allergies.
Medications	None.
Pertinent past medical history	Shoulder injury at age 18 years.
Last oral intake	Unsure of last food intake. Drank beer about an hour before going in the pool.
Events leading up to the injury or illness	The patient was jumping off doing flips from the second-story deck into the above-ground pool when he hit the back of his neck on the bottom of the pool and could not move.

While you are awaiting ALS arrival, you take the time to assess the patient's vital signs **Table 3** and begin a secondary assessment **Table 4**.

Table 3 Daniel's Baseline Vital Signs

Respirations	22 breaths/min and labored
Pulse	55 beats/min and regular
Skin	Cool and moist
Blood pressure	98/68 mm Hg
Oxygen saturation	97% on oxygen

Table 4 Secondary Assessment Findings for Daniel

Level of consciousness	Alert and oriented to person, place, day, and event.
Airway	Intact and patent.
Breathing	Rate is within normal limits but labored.
Circulation	Pulses are present in both upper extremities, but slow.
	Skin below the neck is warm, dry, and flushed.
	Skin on the head is cool, pale, and dry.
Head/neck	Patient is reporting a headache.
	Bruising is noted to forehead.
	No other deformities, contusions, abrasions, punctures, penetrations, paradoxical motion in the chest, burns, tenderness, lacerations, or swelling (DCAP-BTLS) noted on the patient's head or neck.
Chest	No DCAP-BTLS noted to the chest.
	Lung sounds are clear and equal bilaterally with shallow expansion.
Abdomen	Soft, nontender, no rigidity.
Pelvis/genitalia	Pelvis is intact; no deformities or pain on palpation.
	Priapism is noted to the genitalia.
Lower extremities	No DCAP-BTLS or pain noted.
	No movement or sensation in lower extremities.
Upper extremities	No DCAP-BTLS or pain noted.
	No movement or sensation in upper extremities.
Back/neck	Back and neck are unremarkable; no DCAP-BTLS noted to the back when the patient was prone in the pool.
	Patient has neck pain.
	Slight deformity to C4 region noted prior to putting on the collar.
Pain	Unable to rate at this time.
Glasgow coma scale (GCS)	Score: 10 (eye opening, 4; verbal response, 5; motor response, 1).

Before you leave for Camden General Hospital, Alex informs you that ALS has arrived. The paramedic enters the back of the ambulance and asks to be briefed on the patient's situation. After you give her a report, she sets up a bag of saline and attempts to start a large-bore IV in Daniel's left arm.

At this point Daniel is acutely aware of the severity of his injuries and begins to cry. He tells you that in addition to the beer he had consumed earlier in the evening, he also smoked some pot.

Question 4

What type of emotional support do you think this patient needs?

You share with Daniel that there is no way to tell the extent of his injury until he is at the hospital. You reassure him that everything that can be done for him will be. You then reassess his vital signs Table 5.

Table 5 Second Set of Vital Signs for Daniel

Respirations	24 breaths/min and labored
Pulse	52 beats/min and regular
Skin	Flushed, sweaty, cool
Blood pressure	94/62 mm Hg
Oxygen saturation	97% on oxygen

En route to Camden General, the paramedic calls the emergency department staff to notify them of an incoming patient with a possible spinal cord injury. Once you are in the hospital, your patient is immediately assisted to the trauma bay. There is a trauma team waiting for you at bed 1. You and Alex move Daniel to the hospital bed and listen as the paramedic gives an accurate report to the team. They have no further questions for you. You say goodbye to Daniel and wish him the best of luck. Then you head out to wash your hands and start your paperwork. Alex takes the gurney and heads outside to the ambulance to restock and clean up. About 15 minutes later as you are writing your patient care report (PCR), one of the nurses tells you that the radiograph of Daniel's cervical spine shows he fractured C3, C4, and C5. This would explain his paralysis, priapism, and difficulty breathing. You know this will not be an easy recovery for Daniel.

Question 5

What points do you want to make sure to include in your PCR for this patient?

Case Analysis

■ Question 1

What are your scene size-up thoughts for this call?

Given the time of this call, the available light on scene would be one consideration. Is the patient still in the pool? If so, is there a potential for him to drown? What type of pool is it? How did the injury occur? If he is still in the pool, how will you and your crew transfer him out of the pool and secure him to a backboard? Has ALS been dispatched? Are drugs or alcohol involved?

■ Question 2

What is the best way to remove this patient from the pool? What special considerations do you have for securing him to a backboard?

Because the mechanism of injury is significant, with a high probability of spinal cord damage, this patient must be removed from the pool carefully and secured to a backboard. Not only will you and your crew become wet, but the backboard will be wet and slippery. It is imperative to keep the patient warm because his compensatory warming mechanism may not be functioning due to the apparent spinal cord injury.

■ Question 3

What treatment should you initiate before moving him to the ambulance?

Immediately ensure that your patient has a patent airway. Administer high-flow oxygen because your patient is exhibiting signs of difficulty breathing. As mentioned previously, it is critical to keep your patient warm, which would include drying him off and wrapping him with blankets. Finally, ensure that the patient is securely strapped to the backboard and reassess circulation, motor and sensory function, temperature, and pulses every 5 minutes.

■ Question 4

What type of emotional support do you think this patient needs?

Although it is important to be honest with your patient, it is equally important to recognize that you do not have the diagnostic tools to diagnose a spinal cord injury in the field or predict the patient's outcome with any certainty. Acknowledging Daniel's fears and emotions is appropriate, but also maintain a positive attitude that he will receive a definitive diagnosis and continued care at the hospital, where physicians are awaiting his arrival. Sometimes just being there to listen may offer some level of comfort.

Question 5

What points do you want to make sure to include in your PCR for this patient?

As with any PCR, meticulous documentation is essential to good patient care. Specifics should include the following:
- Details of the scene on arrival: where the patient was found, his position, who was assisting him
- The weather (air temperature, conditions, water temperature)
- The approximate height and depth from which he jumped
- Statements the patient made to you and your crew (for example, admitted to drinking beer and smoking pot)
- Statements from witnesses
- Signs and symptoms, including priapism, neurologic deficits, and respiratory difficulty
- How you moved the patient from the pool to the gurney, then to the ambulance
- Documentation of repeat assessment of neurologic status (GCS score, circulation, motor and sensory function, temperature, and pulse)
- Denial of loss of consciousness

Patient Care Report for Daniel

EMS Patient Care Report (PCR)

Date: 07-21-10	Incident No.: 2356	Nature of Call: Possible neck injury	Location: 1468 David Avenue	
Dispatched: 2332	En Route: 2334	At Scene: 2348	Transport: 0004	At Hospital: 0018	In Service: 0045

Patient Information

Age: 21 years	Allergies: No known drug allergies
Sex: Male	Medications: None
Weight (in kg [lb]): 90 kg (200 lb)	Past Medical History: Shoulder injury at age 18 years
	Chief Complaint: Inability to move

Vital Signs

Time	BP	Pulse	Respirations	SpO$_2$
2359	98/68	55 and regular	22 and labored	97% on oxygen
0010	94/62	52 and regular	24 and labored	97% on oxygen

EMS Treatment (circle all that apply)

Oxygen @ <u>15</u> L/min via (circle one): NC (**NRM**) Bag-mask device	Assisted Ventilation	Airway Adjunct	CPR
Defibrillation	Bleeding Control	Bandaging	Splinting	**Other: Immobilization**

Narrative

Dispatched to the scene of a man in swimming pool unable to move. On arrival, patient found in backyard swimming pool, prone in the water, with four friends each holding a limb to keep his head above water. Patient's friends said he was doing flips off the second-floor balcony into the 4-foot above-ground pool. Patient confirmed story and added that he had been drinking beer prior to the incident. Patient was alert and oriented on our arrival and said he was unable to move. Patient denied losing consciousness and his friends confirmed this. Primary assessment revealed a patent airway, shallow breathing with equal expansion and no trauma to the chest. Radial pulses were strong but slow, and skin was pale in the face but flushed to the core and cool and moist. Backboard used to move patient from pool to gurney. Patient was rolled in the water from prone to supine onto the board, which was placed in the water. Patient was removed from the water, dried off, and warmed with blankets. Once patient was out of the water, oxygen therapy was initiated via nonrebreathing mask at 15 L/min. Patient denied any allergies and medications. Patient's only medical history is a right shoulder injury at age 18 years. In the ambulance, patient said he smoked pot earlier in the night. Secondary assessment performed inside the ambulance. Patient remained alert and oriented with an intact airway; breathing was within normal limits but labored, lung sounds clear; pulses present in both upper extremities but slow; skin below neck was warm, dry, and flushed, whereas skin to head was cool, pale, and dry; patient complained of headache, bruising was noted to forehead; abdomen was soft, nontender, and nonrigid; pelvis was intact, no deformities or pain on palpation, priapism was noted to the genitalia; no DCAP-BTLS noted to upper or lower extremities, no movement or sensation to upper or lower extremities, lower extremities were pulseless, and upper extremities had slow palpable pulses; patient was unable to rate pain at that time. GCS score was 10. Paramedic met crew on scene in back of ambulance just prior to leaving for Camden General Hospital. Patient's medical status remained unchanged en route to hospital. Patient care transferred to trauma team without incident.
** End of report**

CASE STUDY 19

Chest Injuries

Man With Open Chest Injuries

It has been a quiet Friday night shift so far. You and your partner, Ella, sit down at the base to watch a movie when a call comes in for a man being beaten in the parking lot of the local comedy club. Ella promptly jumps up and heads for the door while yelling over her shoulder, "Let's go! Sounds like this could be a really bad one!"

Question 1

Prior to arriving at this call, which scene safety factors do you need to take into consideration?

Dispatch instructs you not to enter the scene until law enforcement can secure it.

Question 2

How and where should you establish a staging area?

As you are in the staging area for this call, the dispatcher alerts you that calls are coming in from people in the parking lot indicating that there is a man being hit with a large object, possibly a pipe. Law enforcement is en route.

After the police have cleared the scene, you are notified that it is safe to enter. As you pull into the dark parking lot, you take a careful look around. The police are on scene, and an additional 30 or 40 bystanders are in the parking lot. You drive to the west end of the parking lot, away from the crowd of people, and get out of the ambulance. A police officer walks over to you with a man who is apparently your patient. The man appears to be in his late 20s and is tall and thin. He is wearing jeans and a t-shirt, which have some blood on them. He looks confused. You confirm with police that this is your only patient.

Question 3

How would you proceed with patient assessment?

You introduce yourself and your partner and ask the patient if anything is hurting him. He denies having any pain and starts telling you that people were trying to beat him up in the parking lot. He denies falling or being hit in the head; however, you decide to have the officer hold manual cervical spine stabilization because you are not sure about the reliability of the patient's history. The blood on his t-shirt makes you suspect that he is bleeding from his chest. Ella places the patient on high-flow oxygen, while you expose his chest and shine a flashlight over it. You can see two wounds to the upper right, anterior chest wall. The wounds are small and almost unnoticeable without the benefit of the light.

Question 4

What is the best treatment for an open chest wound?

You immediately advise dispatch that you will need advanced life support (ALS) while Ella pulls the trauma emergency kit off the back of the ambulance. Your patient is oriented, but begins to show signs of combative behavior. You place an occlusive dressing over each of the wounds and move your patient to the controlled environment of the patient compartment in the back of the ambulance. Due to the mechanism of injury and the unreliable patient history, you and your partner apply a cervical collar and full spinal immobilization on a backboard.

Once inside the confines of the patient compartment, you learn that your patient is a 26-year-old named Kyle. He tells you that he was having some drinks while watching the comedy show when he began exchanging angry words with another group. Both he and the other party were escorted out of the building by club security. When they spilled out into the parking lot, a fight broke out. Kyle tells you that he was not hit with a pipe, but that he was stabbed with a small pocket knife and received multiple blows from fists and elbows. It is clear that Kyle's airway is intact. You note that his breathing is shallow and rapid with equal chest expansion and continue with your primary assessment **Table 1**.

Table 1   Primary Assessment Findings for Kyle

General impression	26-year-old man involved in an altercation.
Chief complaint	Pain to the chest.
Level of consciousness	Alert and oriented to person, place, and event.
Airway	Intact.
Breathing	Shallow and rapid, with equal chest expansion.
	Two small incisions to the anterior chest wall.
Circulation	Pulse is strong and regular in both upper extremities.
	Skin is warm, pale, and moist.
Life threats	Open chest wounds.
Pain	No pain reported.
Glasgow coma scale (GCS)	Score: 15 (eye opening, 4; verbal response, 5; motor response, 6).
Interventions	High-flow oxygen.
	Open chest wound covered with occlusive dressings.
	Spinal immobilization initiated.

Due to the mechanism of injury, you assess the rest of Kyle's body in search of any other major wounds. His lower extremities have some red marks on them, but nothing penetrating, and you observe no swelling. You see nothing else that would indicate major injuries anywhere other than on his chest. You ascertain Kyle's baseline vital signs (Table 2) and gather a SAMPLE history, including signs and symptoms, allergies, medications, pertinent past medical history, last oral intake, and events leading up to the injury or illness (Table 3).

Table 2 Baseline Vital Signs for Kyle

Respirations	26 breaths/min and shallow
Pulse	120 beats/min and regular
Skin	Moist, cool, and pale
Blood pressure	118/72 mm Hg
Oxygen saturation	98% on oxygen

Table 3 SAMPLE History for Kyle

Signs and symptoms	Open wounds to the chest from a fight. Pain at injury sights.
Allergies	No known drug allergies.
Medications	None.
Pertinent past medical history	Patient denies any medical history.
Last oral intake	Pizza, chicken wings, and "four to five beers" at the club during the comedy show.
Events leading up to the injury or illness	Fight in the parking lot; attacked by group of people and stabbed with a knife.

Rich, a paramedic, has arrived and is asking for a report on the patient's condition. You fill him in on the patient's history, primary assessment, and vital signs, as the driver begins transport to Chandler Regional Hospital.

Question 5

What complications may be associated with a knife wound to the chest?

Rich has started an IV line with fluids and has the patient on a heart monitor. Remarkably, Kyle's status does not change much en route to the hospital (Table 4). His condition remains stable, but his combative behavior and slurred speech lead you to wonder if he had more alcohol than he admitted. You decide to do a full trauma assessment on Kyle en route to the hospital (Table 5).

Table 4 — Secondary Set of Vital Signs for Kyle

Respirations	24 breaths/min and shallow
Pulse	116 beats/min and regular
Skin	Moist, cool, and pale
Blood pressure	120/74 mm Hg
Oxygen saturation	99% on oxygen

Table 5 — Secondary Assessment Findings for Kyle

Level of consciousness	Remains alert and oriented to person, place, day, and event.
Mechanism of injury	Stab wounds.
Airway	Intact and patent.
Breathing	Difficulty breathing. Pain on inspiration.
Circulation	No major external bleeding. Radial pulses still present and strong. Skin is pale, moist, and cool.
Head/Neck	No pain to the neck. Bruising now apparent to the right corner of the patient's mouth.
Chest	Sternum intact. Occlusive dressing to the wounds are still intact and working well. Lung sounds are clear on the left and diminished on the right.
Abdomen	Abdomen is unremarkable. No pain, distention or deformities, contusions, abrasions, punctures, penetrations, paradoxical motion in the chest, burns, tenderness, lacerations, or swelling (DCAP-BTLS) noted in the abdomen.
Pelvis/Genitalia	Pelvis is intact, no deformities or pain on palpation. Patient denies pain to genitalia region, no priapism noted, and no bleeding to genitalia.
Lower extremities	Pulse, movement, and sensation are present in both lower extremities. Lower extremities have red welt marks, possibly from being struck or kicked. No other DCAP-BTLS noted.
Upper extremities	Pulse, movement, and sensation are present in both upper extremities. Minor lacerations to the palms of both hands.
Back/Neck	Patient denies back and neck pain. No DCAP-BTLS noted.
Pain	Pain to chest is 5 on a scale of 1 to 10.
Pertinent negatives	Patient denies loss of consciousness and denies pain anywhere but his chest.
Glasgow coma scale (GCS)	Score: 15 (eye opening, 4; verbal response, 5; motor response 6).

Question 6

What should be done with the patient's t-shirt once it has been removed to examine his chest for injuries?

Once you are at the hospital and in the trauma bay, you and Rich give your report to the attending physician and nurses. Kyle remains alert despite his potentially life-threatening wounds. As you say good-bye and wish Kyle well, you see a police officer from your district come in the room and ask for any evidence you may have collected during the call. The nurse hands him the red bag containing the patient's t-shirt. You and your crew wash up, take your equipment, and head back out to the ambulance.

Case Analysis

■ Question 1

Prior to arriving at this call, which scene safety factors do you need to take into consideration?

Any dispatched call that comes in as violent or potentially violent warrants police presence. Never assume that you are immune from violence as an EMT. If you are uncertain about whether or not law enforcement has been dispatched to the call, you should ask. Verify this information even before pulling out of your bay or heading toward the call. Always establish a staging area far enough away that you are out of sight of anyone involved in the incident. Only after the police have "cleared" you to approach this scene should you enter. Keep in mind that scene safety is an ongoing consideration. It is important to use your senses (what you hear, see, or smell) throughout the duration of the call.

■ Question 2

How and where should you establish a staging area?

The concept of staging is part of your scene size-up and scene safety assessment. Evaluation of the scene initially begins with the dispatch information. Staging means you will keep your crew and emergency vehicle a safe distance from the call location until law enforcement has cleared you to approach the scene. In the case of violence or potential violence, a safe distance means out of sight of the residence, building, or scene. One reason this is important is because of the possibility that firearms will be discharged.

■ Question 3

How would you proceed with patient assessment?

The patient should be immobilized from a standing position on a backboard with a cervical collar because of the unknown mechanism of injury, slurred speech, combative behavior, and unreliable history. Next, ensure that the patient has an open airway. Place him on high-flow oxygen and examine his chest. If you find open chest wounds, treat them immediately because injuries to the chest may potentially compromise breathing.

Question 4

What is the best treatment for an open chest wound?

External wounds to the body can be deceiving. What looks like a small penetrating wound can actually be very deep. For example, if you do not know the size of the knife or penetrating object that was used, it is almost impossible to tell the extent of the injury. In the case of penetrating wounds or open wounds to the chest, a few key organs are at risk for injury with serious consequences. These organs include the trachea, lungs, heart, and diaphragm. Damage to any of these organs can impede breathing and/or circulation. In addition to breathing and circulatory problems, as much as 1,500 mL of blood can collect in the pleural space of each lung. Any open wounds to the chest are best treated with an occlusive dressing. Occlusive dressings will prevent air from entering the pleural space. Initially, an occlusive dressing can be applied with your gloved hand. This will serve as a temporary occlusive dressing until a more suitable dressing is prepared.

Question 5

What complications may be associated with a knife wound to the chest?

Although the wounds to the patient's chest appear small, you are uncertain about the severity of the injury because you do not know the depth of the knife (or sharp instrument) wounds. Complications associated with chest wounds may include a punctured lung (pneumothorax), tension pneumothorax, hemopneumothorax, severed arteries, contused or lacerated heart, lacerated liver, hemorrhage, and even the potential for spinal cord damage. Any or all of these wounds may significantly impede breathing and circulation.

Question 6

What should be done with the patient's t-shirt once it has been removed to examine his chest for injuries?

If scissors or shears were used to remove the shirt, do not cut through the wound site. Whenever possible, cut along seams or at least cut away from the point of wound entry in the clothing. The shirt, because it is contaminated with blood, should be placed in a red biohazard bag and sealed or tied. Law enforcement officers will want to collect this as evidence. You should turn the patient's property over to the nurse on scene, and the nurse should hand over the shirt to law enforcement. The officers should be told what the bag contains and that there is blood soaked into the clothing.

Patient Care Report for Kyle

EMS Patient Care Report (PCR)

Date: 07-29-2010	Incident No.: 2356	Nature of Call: Possible stabbing		Location: 2225 Sycamore Avenue	
Dispatched: 2250	En Route: 2256	At Scene: 2300	Transport: 2316	At Hospital: 2328	In Service: 2359

Patient Information

Age: 26 years	**Allergies:** No known drug allergies
Sex: Male	**Medications:** None
Weight (in kg [lb]): 88kg (196 lb)	**Past Medical History:** Patient denies
	Chief Complaint: Pain at injury sites

Vital Signs

Time	BP	Pulse	Respirations	SpO$_2$
2315	118/72	120 and regular	26 and shallow	98% on oxygen
2325	120/74	116 and regular	24 and shallow	99% on oxygen

EMS Treatment (circle all that apply)

Oxygen @ **15** L/min via (circle one): NC **(NRM)** Bag-mask Device	Assisted Ventilation	Airway Adjunct	CPR
Defibrillation	Bleeding Control	Bandaging — Occlusive dressing, 4 × 4 dressings	Splinting	**(Other:)** Spinal Immobilization

Narrative

Dispatched for a man involved in a fight in a parking lot. Crew ordered to establish staging area away from the scene until police clear for entry. On arrival to the parking lot, patient presented with disheveled appearance with blood noted on his t-shirt on the chest. Patient placed on high-flow oxygen via nonrebreathing mask. Assessment disclosed two small puncture wounds found to the right upper anterior chest wall. Wounds appear to be approximately 1 cm in diameter and are not bleeding. Wounds were immediately covered with two occlusive dressings. Patient is oriented to place and situation, but is unsure of the time. Patient is immobilized to a backboard for full spinal immobilization including the application of a cervical collar. Once in the ambulance, patient states he was struck in the chest with a small pocket knife and punched in the face several times. Breathing is shallow and rapid with equal expansion. Pulses are strong and regular to both upper extremities; skin is warm, pale, and moist. Detailed assessment reveals the patient is alert and oriented, airway is intact; patient has difficulty breathing with pain on inspiration; no major external bleeding noted. Skin is pale, moist, and cool; radial pulses remain present and strong. No pain noted to the neck; bruising is now visible to the right corner of mouth and right cheek bone. Sternum is intact; occlusive dressing intact on chest wounds, lung sounds clear on the left side and diminished on the right side; abdomen is unremarkable, no pain or distention noted to abdomen. Pelvis is intact and no DCAP-BTLS noted; no priapism or bleeding from genitalia noted; pulse, motor, and sensory functions positive in all four extremities. Red welt marks noted to lower extremities; minor lacerations to the palms of both hands with bleeding controlled with sterile 4″ × 4″ dressings and gauze; pain to chest is rated 5/10; GCS score is 15 throughout treatment and transport. ALS medic 37 present for treatment and transport from the scene. Patient transferred to hospital staff without incident. Red biohazard bag containing patient's t-shirt given to police at the hospital by nursing staff. **End of report**

CASE STUDY 20

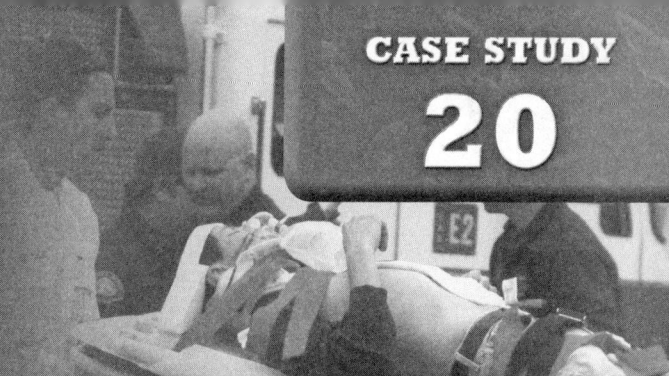

Abdominal and Genitourinary Injuries

Man With Abdominal Pain

It is a cold winter afternoon when you receive a call from the local meat packing plant for a 33-year-old man with abdominal pain. The address is 1224 E. Sioux Avenue and your time out is 1424 hours. You and your partner, Michael, have been to the Bristol Meat Packing plant before, and it is never a pleasant experience. The inside of the building is rather dismal and there is a certain odor in the air that stays with you for hours after you leave.

At the caller's request, you arrive at one of the back loading dock doors and find an employee waiting there for you. As she takes you back to the processing floor, she tells you what is going on with Carlos, your patient. Carlos was working on the processing line using a 25″ meat saw when, for an unknown reason, he fell forward and nearly collapsed to the floor. "When he fell, he landed on his meat saw and it cut into his belly. He is hurt real bad," the woman tells you. You are now aware that this call is much more elaborate than dispatch initially indicated. Michael is already on the radio asking for advanced life support (ALS).

Colleagues have pulled Carlos off of the main processing line and placed him on the floor to the side. This is where you find him lying in a right lateral recumbent position, clutching his belly with blood soaked towels. Despite his naturally olive colored skin, you can tell he looks pale. He is conscious and tracking you as you approach. You introduce yourself and ask him what happened. As he reiterates what his colleague told you previously, it is clear he has a patent airway. He is not displaying any signs of difficulty breathing. You ask a bystander to hold manual cervical in-line stabilization. Michael places the patient on high-flow oxygen via a nonrebreathing mask, while you begin a primary assessment **Table 1**.

Table 1	Primary Assessment Findings for Carlos
Initial general impression	33-year-old man with open abdominal wound.
Chief complaint	Abdominal pain.
Level of consciousness	Alert and oriented to person, place, day, time, and event.
Airway	Patent.
Breathing	Breathing is rapid and equal bilaterally. No trauma to the chest.
Circulation	Skin is pale, moist, and warm. Radial pulse is rapid and strong. Bleeding from open abdominal wound.
Life threats	Abdominal wound/evisceration.
Pain	Abdominal pain rated as 9 on a scale of 1 to 10.

Table 1 Primary Assessment Findings for Carlos (Continued)

Pertinent negatives	Denies hitting head on anything (confirmed by witnesses).
	Denies back and neck pain.
	Denies any shortness of breath or chest pain.
	Denies pain anywhere but his abdomen.
Glasgow coma scale (GCS)	Score: 15 (eye opening, 4; verbal response, 5; motor response, 6).
Interventions	High-flow oxygen applied via nonrebreathing mask.
	Kept patient warm.
	Moistened padded sterile trauma dressings applied.
	Cervical spine precautions and backboard.

Question 1

What specific questions should you ask the patient as you begin your assessment?

Question 2

What would be your treatment priorities for this patient?

Because of the mechanism of injury, you decide it would be best to take full cervical spine precautions at this time. You log roll the patient onto a backboard while Michael carefully secures the patient.

Question 3

How would you treat an abdominal evisceration?

While Michael positions the gurney, you attend to the evisceration, which looks to be about 22 cm in length. There are bowel loops protruding through the wound, and it is apparent why Carlos is in so much pain. After applying a sterile, saline-soaked trauma dressing, you apply and secure a large occlusive dressing. With Carlos now on the gurney, you cover him with two blankets to keep him warm. ALS advises over the radio that they are outside the building and will wait for you to deliver the patient to them.

You use this time to obtain a SAMPLE history from Carlos, including signs and symptoms, allergies, medications, pertinent past medical history, last oral intake, and events leading up to the injury or illness Table 2.

Table 2 — SAMPLE History for Carlos

Signs and symptoms	Severe abdominal pain at site of evisceration, bleeding present upon arrival and then controlled with occlusive and padded dressings.
Allergies	Sulfa drugs.
Medications	None.
Pertinent past medical history	Chronic sinus infections. Bronchitis about 5 weeks ago.
Last oral intake	Lunch around 1130 hours (empanadas, coffee, and a piece of pie).
Events leading up to the injury or illness	Working at station when he felt light-headed and then fell forward onto work station counter top and saw. Possible brief loss of consciousness.

When you load Carlos onto the back of the ambulance, Jennifer, a paramedic, has already set up her equipment and hung a bag of saline in anticipation of starting an IV line.

Question 4

With ALS on board, what is your role as an EMT en route to the hospital?

You begin assessing Carlos's vital signs **Table 3** while Jennifer starts an IV line in his left arm and administers pain medication.

Table 3 — Baseline Vital Signs for Carlos

Respirations	26 breaths/min and regular
Pulse rate	118 beats/min and irregular
Skin	Cool, pale, and moist
Blood pressure	118/72 mm Hg
Oxygen saturation	99% on oxygen

Question 5

If during reassessment you find that the trauma dressing is soaked through, what would be the best course of action?

As Jennifer calls ahead to Sioux Valley Trauma Center to let the trauma team know who you will be bringing in, you perform a secondary assessment on Carlos **Table 4**.

Table 4	Secondary Assessment Findings for Carlos
Level of consciousness	Alert and oriented to person, place, day, and event.
Airway	Intact and patent.
Breathing	Rate is within normal limits.
	No difficulty breathing.
	No pain upon inspiration.
	Lung sounds are clear and equal bilaterally.
	High-flow oxygen administered via a nonrebreathing mask.
Circulation	Pulses present in both upper extremities and remain strong, rapid, and irregular.
	Skin is warm, pale, and moist.
Head/neck	No deformities, contusions, abrasions, punctures, penetrations, paradoxical motion in the chest, burns, tenderness, lacerations, or swelling (DCAP-BTLS) noted on head or neck.
	Patient denies pain to head or neck.
	Pupils are equal, round, regular in size, and react properly to light (PEARRL).
Chest	No DCAP-BTLS noted to chest.
	Lung sounds are clear and equal bilaterally with full expansion.
	Patient denies pain to chest.
Abdomen	Painful evisceration in the lower right quadrant.
	Swelling surrounding the evisceration site.
	Bleeding controlled at injury site with sterile, saline-soaked trauma dressings.
Pelvis/genitalia	Pelvis is intact, no deformities or pain on palpation.
	Patient has some pain to genitalia region, scrotum is beginning to swell, cold packs applied to scrotum to reduce swelling.
Lower extremities	No DCAP-BTLS noted to lower extremities.
	Pulse, movement, and sensation are present in both lower extremities.
Upper extremities	No DCAP-BTLS noted to upper extremities.
	Pulse, movement, and sensation are present in both upper extremities.
Back/neck	No pain/discomfort or DCAP-BTLS noted to back and neck.
Pain	Patient rates his abdominal pain now as 6 out of 10.
	Denies any other pain.
Glasgow coma scale (GCS)	Score: 15 (eye movement, 4; verbal response, 5; motor response, 6).

You take a second set of vital signs on Carlos **Table 5**.

Table 5	Second Set of Vital Signs for Carlos
Respirations	18 breaths/min and regular
Pulse	100 beats/min and irregular
Skin	Cool, pale, and moist
Blood pressure	120/74 mm Hg
Oxygen saturation	99% on oxygen

The 20-minute transport to Sioux Valley Medical Center is uneventful. Jennifer administers pain medication with the fluid replacement and the patient begins to relax slightly. Although Carlos is still in pain, he is not as restless or uncomfortable as he was before. The trauma team greets you at the emergency department entrance and escorts you into the second trauma bay. A supervisor from the Bristol Meat Packing Company is also awaiting your arrival and anxiously asks how Carlos is doing.

Carlos is quickly surrounded by the trauma team. Dr. Cushman asks whether Carlos was conscious when you arrived. You tell him that he was, but that he did say he thinks he lost consciousness when he fell. The physician gives you a nod of approval, "Good job." After washing your hands and gathering your equipment, you head back to the ambulance.

Case Analysis

■ **Question 1**

What specific questions should you ask the patient as you begin your assessment?

It is important to determine whether the patient lost consciousness—either prior to, during, or after the fall. It is also important to ask the patient what happened, or what caused the fall. Could this also be a medical call? As you begin to investigate what happened, it is crucial to keep an open mind and think critically about the possible causes of your patient's trauma.

■ **Question 2**

What would be your treatment priorities for this patient?

Because you have already determined that the patient has an open airway, make sure that his breathing is adequate, examine his chest to check for signs of DCAP-BTLS, apply high-flow oxygen, hold manual cervical spine stabilization, and control any bleeding. Remember: if you find any life threats during your primary assessment, treat those immediately.

■ Question 3

How would you treat an abdominal evisceration?

It is vital that every attempt be made to avoid further damage to the abdominal organs as long as they are out of the abdominal cavity to ensure their viability for surgical replacement. When the organs are inside the body they are constantly bathed in body fluids to ensure moistness. Therefore, it is crucial to keep those same organs moist during treatment and transport to definitive care. It may be necessary to remoisten the trauma dressings en route to the hospital depending on the length of transport.

Cut away any clothing on and around the wound. Abdominal eviscerations are best treated with sterile, saline-soaked, large trauma dressings (10 x 30, for example). Tape the dressing in place. Treat the patient for shock (administer high-flow oxygen, keep the patient warm, and reassess and monitor vital signs).

■ Question 4

With ALS on board, what is your role as an EMT en route to the hospital?

You should remain an active participant in the care of this patient, working together closely with ALS to ensure excellent patient care is provided. Assessing the patient's vital signs and performing a secondary assessment are all part of the EMT's responsibilities, whether or not you are working with ALS personnel.

■ Question 5

If during reassessment you find that the trauma dressing is soaked through, what would be the best course of action?

Dressings that you used to take care of a patient's bleeding that become soaked through should have more sterile dressings added to them. Do not remove the dressings that you have applied because removing them may cause bleeding to worsen or release clots/emboli that could travel into the patient's blood stream and create further problems.

Man With Abdominal Pain

Patient Care Report for Carlos

EMS Patient Care Report (PCR)

Date: 01-29-11	Incident No.: 1124		Nature of Call: Abdominal injury		Location: 1224 E. Sioux Avenue
Dispatched: 1424	En Route: 1425	At Scene: 1436	Transport: 1450	At Hospital: 1518	In Service: 1532

Patient Information

Age: 33 years	Allergies: Sulfa drugs
Sex: Male	Medications: None
Weight (in kg [lb]): 65kg (145lb)	Past Medical History: Chronic sinus infections, bronchitis 5 weeks ago
	Chief Complaint: Abdominal pain

Vital Signs

Time: 1441	BP: 118/72	Pulse: 118 and irregular	Respirations: 26 and regular	SpO_2: 99% on oxygen
Time: 1453	BP: 120/74	Pulse: 100 and irregular	Respirations: 18 and regular	SpO_2: 99% on oxygen
Time:	BP:	Pulse:	Respirations:	SpO_2:

EMS Treatment
(circle all that apply)

Oxygen @ <u>15</u> L/min via (circle one): NC (NRM) Bag-mask Device	Assisted Ventilation	Airway Adjunct	CPR
Defibrillation (Bleeding Control)	(Bandaging) Occlusive dressing Trauma dressing	Splinting	(Other:) Spinal Immobilization Cold Packs Warming

Narrative

Dispatched for a man with abdominal pain. On arrival, crew met by employee at loading dock door who led us to the patient. Patient found lying on the floor in a right lateral recumbent position, alert to crew. Patient's airway is patent, with no visible signs of difficulty breathing. Manual spinal stabilization is initiated due to the fall from the packing line. Patient administered high-flow oxygen via a nonrebreathing mask. No trauma is found to the chest. Skin is pale, moist, and warm; radial pulses are present and rapid and strong. Bleeding can be seen from the open abdominal wound. Pain to the abdomen is rated a 9/10. Patient denies hitting his head, denies back and neck pain, denies shortness of breath, and denies any pain other than pain to the abdomen. On assessment of the patient's abdomen, an abdominal evisceration is noted to the lower right quadrant with bowel protrusion. Evisceration is immediately bandaged with a sterile saline soaked trauma dressing. Blankets applied to patient for warmth. Patient immobilized to backboard and moved to gurney. Medic 52 meets crew on board ambulance for ALS care and treatment. Secondary assessment reveals the patient remains alert and oriented. Patient's airway remains intact; breathing rate is within normal limits, no difficulty breathing, no pain on inspiration, lung sounds clear and equal bilaterally. Oxygen therapy administered throughout duration of transport. Strong pulses remain in upper extremities; skin is warm, pale, and moist; no DCAP-BTLS noted to the head/neck region. Patient continues to deny pain or discomfort to the head/neck region; PEARRL; no DCAP-BTLS noted to the chest; lung sounds clear; evisceration in lower right quadrant with swelling present in area; pelvis intact, no DCAP-BTLS, no pain on palpation, swelling noted to scrotum en route to hospital; cold packs applied to area to help reduce swelling; no DCAP-BTLS noted to upper or lower extremities; pulses are strong and present in all four extremities. After ALS administered pain medication, patient reported pain of 6/10 en route to hospital. GCS score remains 15 for duration of treatment and transport to Sioux Valley Medical Center. Patient transferred to hospital staff without incident. **End of report**

CASE STUDY 21

Musculoskeletal Injuries

Woman With a Leg Injury

It is a cold February morning in your hometown of Wolcott, Vermont, when you receive a call for a woman who fell off of a horse and injured her leg. While Allen, your driver, confirms the address, you look up the location in your map book. En route to the call you discuss the fact that neither one of you has ever been to this horse stable, although you have both heard of it and have probably driven by it many times over the years. Time out for the call is 0846 hours.

Question 1

What equipment do you anticipate you will need for this call?

You arrive on location approximately 7 minutes after receiving the call. Upon entering the grounds of the stables, you note how bumpy the ride in the ambulance is due to the packed mud and snow. An employee of the stable guides you to the correct building and your partner parks the ambulance. As you are gathering equipment, you wonder how you will move the patient from the dirt floor of the riding stable to the location of the parked ambulance. The horses in the riding ring are all calm, held in control by other riders, and far away from your injured patient.

You find a woman lying on the loosely packed dirt floor of the riding stable in full riding gear—a heavy riding coat, leather gloves, and fully insulated riding pants. She is found in a supine position with blankets under her head and covering her shivering body. The estimated temperature in the riding stable is about 33°F, but the wind is blocked from the enclosure. Loosely packed dirt is found on the patient, under the patient, and on the equipment that is set down.

Question 2

What considerations should you make for the patient because of the outdoor temperature?

You introduce yourself to the patient and find out that her name is Kim and that she is 26 years old. Kim is alert and oriented to person, place, day, and time.

Question 3

What questions would you initially ask the patient to determine the chief complaint and the extent of her injury?

The patient denies losing consciousness, which is confirmed by witnesses. As your partner begins to stabilize her head and neck, you quickly ask Kim further questions. She denies striking and injuring her head or neck. She tells you that her horse reared and she tumbled off and landed on her left leg. She said she heard a "crunching" sound when she landed and is pretty certain she broke her leg. "Almost all of my weight landed on my left leg when I fell," Kim tells you. Another rider who witnessed the fall came over to her and immediately took control of Kim's horse. She is unable to move her left leg and is in pain.

Kim's airway is intact and clear and her breathing appears normal. She denies having any breathing complaints or difficulties. Due to the cold temperatures, you defer examining her chest and upper body until after moving her to the warmth of the ambulance. You do not find any obvious bleeding as you do your best to inspect through the dense clothing and dirt. Kim continues to complain only of lower left leg pain. You tell her that you will need to expose her leg to stabilize it before moving her.

Question 4

How would you stabilize the patient's leg injury?

Fortunately, her insulated riding pants have zippers on the side. You unzip them all the way up to the groin and find that she is wearing a pair of denim jeans underneath the riding pants. You tell Kim that you will need to cut the jeans to fully expose her injured leg for assessment. You cut her jeans along the seam to gain access to her injured leg. Once her leg is exposed, you immediately see a large swollen area next to her tibia at the midpoint. The area has already started to bruise and it appears that a bone fragment is protruding into the skin, although not completely through it. The patient rates her pain as an 8 on a scale of 1 to 10 and describes it as sharp. You ask Allen to see if advanced life support (ALS) is available to provide pain relief for your patient and place her on high-flow oxygen via a nonrebreathing mask.

You perform a primary assessment on Kim before packaging for transport **Table 1**.

Table 1 Primary Assessment Findings for Kim

General impression	26-year-old woman with possible fracture to lower left leg.
Chief complaint	Lower left leg pain.
Level of consciousness	Alert and oriented to person, place, day, time, and event.
Airway	Patent.
Breathing	Breathing rate is within normal limits.
	No trauma noted to the chest.
Circulation	Skin is pale, cool, and dry.
	Radial pulse is rapid and strong.
	No bleeding noted.
Life threats	No life threats noted during primary assessment.

Table 1	Primary Assessment Findings for Kim (Continued)
Pain	Lower left leg pain rated as 8 on a scale of 1 to 10.
Pertinent negatives	No difficulty breathing, no pain other than at injury site. No loss of consciousness.
Glasgow coma scale (GCS)	Score: 15 (eye opening, 4; verbal response, 5; motor response, 6).
Interventions	High-flow oxygen applied via a nonrebreathing mask. Blankets given to keep patient warm. Left leg stabilized until further assessment.

You begin to splint Kim's injured leg with padded splints and cravats. You also place a wrapped cold pack on her injury site to help relieve some of the pain. You decide to move her with a scoop stretcher because it will alleviate the need to roll her onto a backboard. Once she is secured to the scoop stretcher, each responder—you, Allen, and two fire fighters who heard the call and stopped by to offer assistance—takes a corner of the scoop stretcher and carefully walks to the gurney outside of the riding arena. Once the patient is inside the warm ambulance, you remove her coat to accurately obtain a blood pressure and full set of vital signs Table 2.

Table 2	Baseline Vital Signs for Kim
Respirations	18 breaths/min and regular
Pulse	100 beats/min and regular
Skin	Pale, cool, and dry
Blood pressure	120/78 mm Hg
Oxygen saturation	99% on oxygen

After you assess Kim's vital signs and find them stable and within normal limits, you continue with a SAMPLE history, including signs and symptoms, allergies, medications, pertinent past medical history, last oral intake, and the events leading up to the injury or illness Table 3.

Table 3	SAMPLE History for Kim
Signs and symptoms	Swollen, deformed, painful lower left leg. Sharp pain 8 out of 10 at injury site.
Allergies	Penicillin.
Medications	Birth control pills (Ortho-Novum).
Pertinent past medical history	None.
Last oral intake	Toasted bagel with butter and a cup of coffee at about 0730 hours.
Events leading up to the injury or illness	Riding her horse when he reared up and she fell off, landing on her left leg.

Allen comes back to the rear compartment and tells you that ALS intercept for pain control is not currently available. You thank him for the information and indicate that it is time to head to the hospital. Kim tells you that she would prefer to be transported to Copley Hospital, which is about a 25-minute ride from your location. You agree that transport there would be a good choice because Kim's primary care physician is affiliated with the hospital and it is one of the closest trauma facilities.

Question 5

How will you continue to assess your patient's condition en route to the hospital?

With Kim's leg stabilized in the back of the warm, moving ambulance, you begin your secondary assessment **Table 4**. You complete a head-to-toe exam and find no new injuries, other than some minor abrasions to the palms of her hands. You also reassess her pain and vital signs now that her leg is immobilized and ice has been applied **Table 5**. She says the pain is now throbbing and is a 6 out of 10. She still has a pulse, movement, and sensation in all four extremities.

Table 4 Secondary Assessment Findings for Kim

Level of consciousness	Alert and oriented to person, place, day, and event.
Airway	Intact and patent.
Breathing	Rate is within normal limits.
	No difficulty breathing.
	No pain upon inspiration.
	Lung sounds are clear and equal bilaterally.
	High-flow oxygen administered via a nonrebreathing mask.
Circulation	Pulses present in both upper extremities and remain strong and regular.
	Skin is warm, pale, and dry.
Head/neck	No deformities, contusions, abrasions, punctures, penetrations, paradoxical motion in the chest, burns, lacerations, tenderness, or swelling (DCAP-BTLS) noted to the head or neck.
	Patient denies pain to head or neck.
	Pupils are equal, round, regular in size, and react properly to light (PEARRL).
Chest	No DCAP-BTLS noted to chest.
	Lung sounds are clear and equal bilaterally with full expansion.
	Patient denies pain to chest.
Abdomen	Soft and non-tender to touch, no pain, swelling, or rigidity noted upon assessment.
Pelvis/genitalia	Pelvis is intact, no deformities or pain on palpation.
	Assessment deferred because patient denies any injury or pain to genitalia.

Table 4 — Secondary Assessment Findings for Kim (Continued)

Lower extremities	Right lower extremity is without pain or DCAP-BTLS.
	Pulse, motor, and sensory functions are all positive.
	Left lower extremity is painful with swelling, deformity, and tenderness at mid-shaft tibia area.
Upper extremities	No DCAP-BTLS noted to upper extremities.
	Pulse, movement, and sensation are present in both upper extremities.
Back/neck	No pain/discomfort or DCAP-BTLS noted to back and neck.
Pain	Patient rates left leg pain as 6 out of 10.
	Denies any other pain.
Glasgow coma scale (GCS)	Score: 15 (eye opening, 4; verbal response, 5; motor response, 6).

Table 5 — Second Set of Vital Signs for Kim

Respirations	14 breaths/min and regular
Pulse	88 beats/min and regular
Skin	Warm and dry
Blood pressure	118/74 mm Hg
Oxygen saturation	100% on oxygen

Kim remains alert, oriented, and talkative en route to the hospital. On arrival at the emergency department, you are instructed to move Kim to bed 3L in the trauma bay. You immediately transfer Kim with the bed railings up, bed down in the lowest position, and blanket on. As you turn to wash your hands at the sink, you wish Kim well with her injury and recovery.

Case Analysis

■ Question 1

What equipment do you anticipate you will need for this call?

In addition to the standard equipment that should be brought to the patient on each call (fully stocked medic bag, oxygen, bag-mask device, and automated external defibrillator), you should bring the splints you carry on your truck or ambulance with you (padded splints, formable splints, vacuum, or traction) based on the dispatch information.

Question 2

What considerations should you make for the patient because of the outdoor temperature?

Warmth! It is imperative to keep your patient warm. The climate of the riding ring is cold. The cold environment, combined with the fact that Kim has been lying on the ground unable to move, makes her more prone to hypothermia (less movement means slower blood circulation throughout the body). Blankets and a warm patient care compartment are necessary to ensure this patient stays comfortable and free of hypothermic complications.

Question 3

What questions would you initially ask the patient to determine the chief complaint and the extent of her injury?

It is essential to determine whether Kim lost consciousness after the fall. It is also important to know if Kim hit her head or neck during the fall. Losing consciousness or hitting her head could indicate a traumatic brain injury or concussion. Hitting her neck during the fall could indicate a potential spinal cord injury. What else is causing her pain? If witnesses are available, it is important to verify the history of the event with them.

Question 4

How would you stabilize the patient's leg injury?

Because Kim has a closed wound, you do not need to bandage an open injury at the fracture site. With the skin still intact, her chances of infection are lower. While your partner stabilizes the injured extremity, assess pedal pulses, movement, and sensation in the injured leg prior to applying any splinting devices. Clothing to the injury site should be removed so you have adequate access for a full assessment of the damaged extremity. Any number of commercially available splinting devices may be used to stabilize this injury as long as the goals of splinting are met: stabilize the adjacent joints above and below the injury site.

Question 5

How will you continue to assess your patient's condition en route to the hospital?

Given that you have a commute time of about 25 minutes, you will most likely have time to perform a secondary assessment as well as a reassessment. Even though Kim appears to have an isolated extremity injury, it would be best, given her mechanism of injury, to assess her more thoroughly from head-to-toe en route to the hospital. During your assessment of Kim, be sure to recheck your interventions as well. Does she still have pulses, movement, and sensation in her injured leg? What is her pain level? Has the pain radiated? Has the pain changed? Has pain or discomfort developed anywhere else on your patient? Is there DCAP-BTLS anywhere else on her body? Is she maintaining her level of alertness?

Patient Care Report for Kim

EMS Patient Care Report (PCR)

Date: 02-21-2010	Incident No.: 12151	Nature of Call: Fall from horse		Location: 751 Browncroft Blvd.	
Dispatched: 0846	En Route: 0846	At Scene: 0853	Transport: 0915	At Hospital: 0946	In Service: 1005

Patient Information

Age: 26 years	**Allergies:** Penicillin
Sex: Female	**Medications:** Birth control pills (Ortho-Novum)
Weight (in kg [lb]): 65 kg (145 lb)	**Past Medical History:** None
	Chief Complaint: Lower left leg pain

Vital Signs

Time	BP	Pulse	Respirations	SpO$_2$
0910	120/78	100 and regular	18 and regular	99% on oxygen
0927	118/74	88 and regular	14 and regular	100% on oxygen

EMS Treatment (circle all that apply)

Oxygen @ <u>15</u> L/min via (circle one): NC **(NRM)** Bag-mask Device	Assisted Ventilation	Airway Adjunct	CPR
Defibrillation	Bleeding Control	Bandaging	**(Splinting)**	**(Other:)** Warming Cold packs

Narrative

Dispatched for a woman who fell from a horse with a leg injury. On arrival, crew escorted into the dirt floor riding ring to find 26-year-old woman lying supine on the ground, alert to crew and surroundings. Horse had been secured by another rider. Patient denies hitting head or neck during fall from horse. Patient denies losing consciousness, which is confirmed by a fellow rider who witnessed the fall. Patient describes how her horse reared up and she lost her grip on the reigns and fell to the dirt-packed ground, landing with almost all her weight on her left leg. Patient's chief complaint is pain to her lower left leg. Patient's airway is intact on arrival with no apparent obstructions. Patient's respirations are unlabored. Rapid scan for blood finds no external bleeding or blood-soaked clothing. Skin is cool, pale, and dry. Assessment of injured leg reveals a painful, swollen, tender lower left extremity, with bone protruding to the skin surface, but not through it. Pain rated as 8/10 at this time. Lower left leg is immobilized using padded splints and cravats. Cold packs help relieve pain at the injury site. Two wool blankets applied to patient for warmth. Patient placed on high-flow oxygen via a nonrebreathing mask. ALS is called for pain control, but is not available. A posterior pedal pulse is present but weak in her left leg, movement is diminished and sensation is positive prior to securing padded splint to injured leg. Patient moved from ground using a scoop stretcher and walked out of riding ring to gurney near parked ambulance. Patient requests transport to Copley Hospital. Secondary assessment reveals that the patient is alert and oriented with airway intact; breathing is within normal limits, lung sounds are clear and equal bilaterally, and patient's breathing is free from difficulty and pain. Strong pulses are present in both upper extremities; no bleeding noted on body. Skin is warm, pale, and dry; no DCAP-BTLS noted on head, neck, chest, right lower extremity, and upper extremities. Patient denies feeling dizzy or light-headed, denies any pain to chest. Abdomen is soft and non-tender and free of swelling or pain. Pelvis is intact and without pain. Right lower extremity is without pain; pulses, motor, and sensory functions are all positive; left lower extremity is painful (6/10) with swelling now noted to the mid-shaft tibia. Movement is diminished and sensation is present; discomfort and deformity is noted to the back and neck; GCS score is 15 en route to Copley Hospital. Patient is triaged and transferred to bed 3L in the trauma bay. Patient moved to bed and scoop stretcher removed. Bed rails raised, bed lowered. **End of report**

CASE STUDY 22

Environmental Emergencies

Man With Hyperthermia

It is an unusually sunny, hot, and humid October morning for the Chicago Marathon. The runners have all taken their spots at the starting line. The weatherman reports the temperature to be 80°F with the humidity at 75% and expected to climb to 90%. "There must be over 1,000 participants," you say to your partner, Paul. This is the second year in a row that you and Paul have been assigned to the marathon as one of the many emergency medical service (EMS) crews on standby. You can't help but wonder how many will make it to the finish line. Nearly 2 hours into the race you are called over the radio by the EMS operations director. They need you to bring the ambulance over to the medical tent for a patient who is ill and will need transport to the hospital for further evaluation.

Question 1

What concerns do you have for runners on a day like today?

You arrive in the medical tent to find three EMTs surrounding a runner with fans circulating on him. His name is Carl. He is 53 years old and has a runner's build, thin and muscular. He is lying in a left lateral recumbent position on the cot and barely able to speak. His face is bright red, and hot to the touch, but he is not sweating. Finn, one of the EMTs, tells you that Carl had just finished the half-marathon (13.1 miles) when he walked over to the tent for some cool air and fluids. As Carl began drinking his sports drink, he got a glazed look on his face. That is when the medical staff assisted him to a cot and sat him down. When the patient nearly lost consciousness, they called you for transport to the hospital.

After telling Carl who you are, you ask him how he is feeling. His eyes are open, but he looks very confused. He mumbles something incoherent and then becomes unresponsive. You open his airway and find that he is breathing so you immediately apply high-flow oxygen via a nonrebreathing mask, and expose his chest to check his breathing further. You do not note any signs of trauma to the chest. As you touch his skin you, again, note that he is very hot. Radial pulses are weak and thready. His carotid pulse is currently weak and rapid. His skin remains flushed despite the use of fans. There are no signs of bleeding or trauma on his body. You complete your primary assessment Table 1.

Environmental Emergencies

Table 1 — Primary Assessment Findings for Carl

General impression	53-year-old man, unresponsive and extremely hot to the touch.
Chief complaint	Unresponsive.
Level of consciousness	Unresponsive.
Airway	Manually opened airway with head tilt–chin lift maneuver.
Breathing	Shallow.
Circulation	Hot, flushed, and dry skin. Carotid pulse is weak and thready.
Life threats	Possible heat stroke.
Pertinent Negatives	No chest trauma. No bleeding.
Pupils	Sluggish.
Glasgow coma scale (GCS)	Score: 7 (eye opening, 2; verbal response, 4; motor response, 1).
Interventions	High-flow oxygen applied via a nonrebreathing mask. Opened airway with head tilt–chin lift maneuver. Active cooling methods.

Question 2

What other assessment tool could you use to evaluate the severity of Carl's condition?

After your partner returns from the rig with the thermometer, you take the patient's axillary temperature. You are shocked when it registers at 105°F. You reset the thermometer and take his temperature again with the same result. His core temperature could very well be one to two degrees higher than this. The patient's temperature is alarming. It is time to transport Carl to the hospital. You ask the medical tent staff to call for ALS. They tell you the three ALS providers who were on stand-by for the event are attending to other patients on the race course at the moment.

Question 3

What is happening to Carl's thermoregulatory mechanisms?

Question 4

What are your treatment priorities for Carl?

Paul has brought the gurney over, and with the help of the medical tent staff, you transfer Carl to the awaiting gurney. Wrapped cold packs have been applied to Carl's armpits, groin, and the back of his knees and neck. His shirt, shoes, and socks have been removed and you ask Finn to rapidly fan Carl as you wheel him out to the ambulance. Once on board the rig, you get the mister out of the cabinet and ask Finn if he can start misting Carl while you obtain a set of baseline vital signs **Table 2**. Finn says he would be happy to help and can go with you to the hospital. Paul confirms that you want to go to Chicago General, which is only about 10 blocks away, and the rig pulls out in "red" mode utilizing lights and sirens.

Table 2 Baseline Vital Signs for Carl

Respirations	32 breaths/min, rapid and shallow
Pulse	108 beats/min, weak and irregular
Skin	Hot, flushed, and dry
Blood pressure	98/60 mm Hg
Oxygen saturation	88% on high-flow oxygen

Question 5

What are your treatment priorities based on Carl's vital signs?

Michael yells back and asks if you would like him to call ahead to Chicago General for you. "Yes. Tell them our patient's GCS is 7, temp of 105, and we are assisting ventilations of a 53-year-old man who just ran the half marathon." "Got it," Michael responds. Finn continues to cool the patient actively while you begin to assist ventilations with a bag-mask device.

It is a busy day at Chicago General. Several ambulances are in the emergency department (ED) parking lot. As you approach the ED doors you see a long triage line in front of you. Fortunately, for your patient, the ED staff has been notified and is awaiting your arrival. They quickly usher you into the resuscitation bay. As you transfer Carl over to the hospital bed you quickly update the staff on his condition and treatment. With Carl in the competent hands of the ED staff, you, Paul, and Finn take your equipment, wash up, and head to the rig.

Case Analysis

From 1979 to 2003 (the latest statistics available), 8,015 deaths in the United States were heat related, with 48% of the deaths due to weather conditions. Heat-related illnesses can affect many groups of people in a variety of industries and recreations **Table 3**.

Table 3	Populations Most Susceptible to Heat-Related Illnesses
People involved in vigorous activity in hot weather, such as running, hiking, cycling, and rock climbing	
Adults older than 65 years	
Infants and young children	
People who are: • Obese • On certain medications • Not acclimated to the heat • Have chronic illnesses	
Employees in specific industries or working environments, such as: • Roofing • Road repair • Construction • Farming operations (including crop workers) • Iron and steel foundries • Brick firing and ceramics operations • Glass products manufacturing plants • Boiler room operators • Fire fighters, EMS employees, law enforcement • Restaurant kitchens • Bakeries • Engine rooms • Dam and bridge builders	

■ Question 1

What concerns do you have for runners on a day like today?

The ambient air temperature, as well as the humidity, is a concern for not only runners but also anyone who is exposed to this environment. The body attempts to maintain homeostasis (equilibrium in the normal physiologic states of the body). Like homeostasis, thermoregulation is another way the body attempts to maintain balance. The thermoregulation mechanism in the body strives to keep the body's temperature at 98.6°F (37°C). When outside temperatures are at extremes, it becomes more difficult for the body to maintain homeostasis. The body generates heat through activity, such as breathing, moving, eating, and digestion. Just as the body generates heat, the body also needs to counterbalance by getting rid of excess heat Figure 1. There are five different ways in which the body transfers heat Table 4.

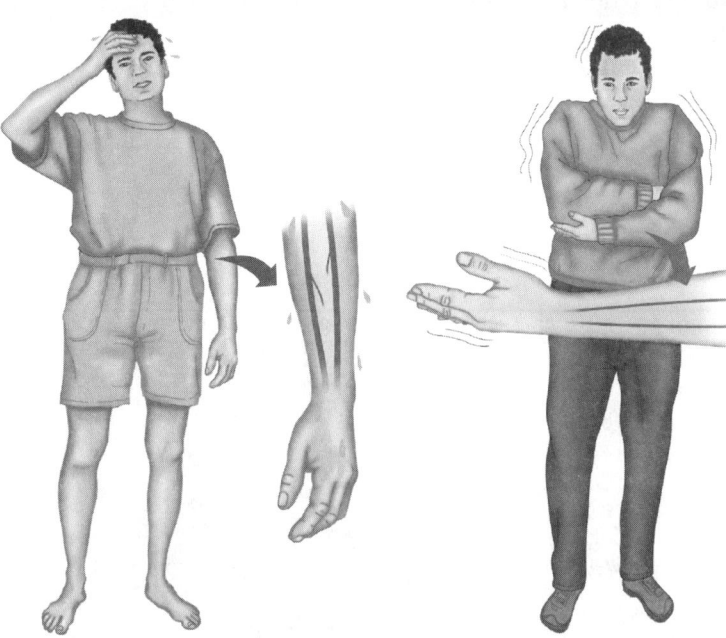

Hot Environment
- Blood vessels dilate, maximizing heat loss from skin
- Body sweats, causing evaporation and cooling

Body temperature decreases

Cold Environment
- Blood vessels constrict, minimizing heat loss from skin
- Muscles shiver, generating heat

Body temperature increases

Figure 1 Body mechanisms work to maintain a constant internal temperature, regardless of the ambient temperature.

Table 4 Ways in Which the Body Transfers Heat

Method of Heat Transfer	Definition	Example
Conduction	The transfer of heat by direct contact.	Holding an ice cube causes it to melt.
Convection	The transfer of heat through circulating air.	Food cooking in an oven.
Evaporation	The conversion of a liquid to a gas, which requires energy.	Swimmers who do not dry off become cold after leaving the water.
Radiation	The transfer of heat by radiant energy.	Placing your hands over a fire will warm them.
Respiration	Body heat is lost as warm air from the body is exhaled and cold air from the atmosphere is inhaled. Heat can be gained in hot environments.	A runner, who breathes more heavily and deeply as he or she runs, will become overheated in a hot environment.

In this scenario, the ability of the patient to lose heat to cool the body is hampered by the high ambient air temperature (which impedes radiation) and high humidity (which impedes evaporation). The higher the percentage of relative humidity, the higher the risk of heat stroke, or even death Figure 2.

NOAA's National Weather Service
Heat Index

Temperature (°F) →	80	82	84	86	88	90	92	94	96	98	100	102	104	106	108	110
Relative Humidity (%)																
40	80	81	83	85	88	91	94	97	101	105	109	114	119	124	130	136
45	80	82	84	87	89	93	96	100	104	109	114	119	124	130	137	
50	81	83	85	88	91	95	99	103	108	113	118	124	131	137		
55	81	84	86	89	93	97	101	106	112	117	124	130	137			
60	82	84	88	91	95	100	105	110	116	123	129	137				
65	82	85	89	93	98	103	108	114	121	126	130					
70	83	86	90	95	100	105	112	119	126	134						
75	84	88	92	97	103	109	116	124	132							
80	84	89	94	100	106	113	121	129								
85	85	90	96	102	110	117	126	135								
90	86	91	98	105	113	122	131									
95	86	93	100	108	117	127										
100	87	95	103	112	121	132										

Likelihood of Heat Disorders with Prolonged Exposure or Strenuous Activity

☐ Caution ■ Extreme Caution ■ Danger ■ Extreme Danger

Figure 2 The National Oceanic and Atmospheric Administration's National Weather Service Heat Index Chart.

Question 2

What other assessment tool could you use to evaluate the severity of Carl's condition?

A thermometer will help you determine the severity of the patient's condition. Hyperthermia is defined as a core body temperature of 101°F (38.4°C) or above. If your patient had a core body temperature of 100°F (38°C) the severity of his condition may not be as grave as it is with a core body temperature of 105°F (41°C).

Question 3

What is happening to Carl's thermoregulatory mechanisms?

Carl's thermoregulatory mechanisms are no longer able to compensate and rid the body of excess heat. This patient requires swift, active cooling. When the thermoregulatory system ceases to work it is a true emergency.

Question 4

What are your treatment priorities for Carl?

Maintaining the ABCs and active cooling are crucial to the survival of your patient. Active cooling involves:
- Removing clothing from the patient
- Moving the patient to a cooler environment, if possible (shade, air-conditioned building or ambulance)
- Cool/cold packs to the groin, axillary, and back of the neck
- Active fanning, preferably with a mister (misting water while fanning the patient)

Question 5

What are your treatment priorities based on Carl's vital signs?

This patient needs aggressive airway and breathing support. A nasopharyngeal airway (NPA) could be inserted to help maintain the airway. Because the patient is hyperventilating at a rate of 32 breaths/min and has a decreased level of consciousness and poor tidal volume, he will need assisted ventilations en route to the hospital.

Patient Care Report for Carl

EMS Patient Care Report (PCR)

Date: 10-04-2010	Incident No.: 3421	Nature of Call: Illness	Location: Congress Avenue and First Street	
Dispatched: 1006	En Route: 1006	At Scene: 1007	Transport: 1017	At Hospital: 1029	In Service: 1100

Patient Information

Age: 53 years	Allergies: Unknown
Sex: Male	Medications: Unknown
Weight (in kg [lb]): 92kg (165lb)	Past Medical History: Unknown
	Chief Complaint: Unresponsive

Vital Signs

Time: 1015	BP: 98/60	Pulse: 108, weak and irregular	Respirations: 32, rapid and shallow	SpO$_2$: 88% on oxygen
Time:	BP:	Pulse:	Respirations:	SpO$_2$:
Time:	BP:	Pulse:	Respirations:	SpO$_2$:

EMS Treatment
(circle all that apply)

Oxygen @ 15 L/min via (circle one): NC **NRM** **Bag-mask device**	**Assisted Ventilation**	**Airway Adjunct** NPA	CPR
Defibrillation	Bleeding Control	Bandaging	Splinting	**Other:** Active Cooling

Narrative

On standby at the Chicago Marathon when we were dispatched to the medical tent for a male who was feeling ill. After arriving at the medical tent, patient was found left lateral recumbent on a cot with 3 EMTs present and fanning patient. EMTs reported that patient finished the half marathon when he walked to the medical tent for fluids and a cool spot to sit down. The patient was given a sports drink and then became dazed and his eyes glazed over. Crew immediately sat patient down on cot. According to medical tent staff, patient almost lost consciousness, which is when they called for an EMS transport. Crew attempted to get a response from patient, although his eyes were open, he did not respond with any coherent words. Patient then became unresponsive. Airway manually opened using the head tilt-chin lift and a nonrebreathing mask is applied. No trauma noted to his chest, breathing was rapid and shallow; skin was very hot, dry, and flushed in the face, no bleeding present, radial pusles were weak and thready. An axillary temperature was assessed using a digital thermometer and reveals a temp of 105 °F. Patient immediately transferred to the gurney. Cold packs were applied to the armpits, groin, back of knees, and back of neck. Shirt, shoes, socks were removed. Crew member fanned patient while moving to the ambulance. Patient was misted and fanned en route to the hospital. Patient's ventilations were assisted en route to Chicago General due to the rapid, shallow rate. GCS was 7. Due to the crew assisting ventilations and doing active cooling methods, there was no time to perform a secondary assessment. ALS was not available so we drove directly to Chicago General. Patient was transferred to ED staff, bed 3 in the trauma bay. **End of report**

Obstetrics and Neonatal Care

CASE STUDY 23

Woman in Labor in a Car

It is a cold, snowy, winter evening in January as your driver, Marty, backs the rig up into the ambulance bay. As you are preparing to end your shift for the night, a call comes in for a woman in labor at a coffee shop a few blocks from your base. Fire first response has been dispatched. Their station is located one block from the call location. You request ALS for this call in case there are any complications. The dispatcher lets you know that due to the inclement weather, ALS is approximately 20 minutes away from the scene. Time out is 2333 hours.

You arrive on scene within 3 minutes to find a car parked haphazardly in front of the coffee shop. There is a small crowd gathered around the front passenger side of the car. As you approach, you can see that the passenger door is open and EMT fire fighter Preston is kneeling with a newborn in his arms, suctioning the airway. The cord is still attached. You get closer and now see the mother sitting in the passenger seat with a look of awe and dismay on her face. Behind you stands the driver of the car, your patient's husband. He stopped the car to go into the coffee shop to call for an ambulance when his wife indicated that birth was imminent.

Question 1

What questions would you ask during your primary assessment on this patient? What concerns do you have for the mother and newborn?

EMT fire fighter Preston has suctioned the airway, clamped the cord, and is now cutting it. You wait behind him with a large cotton blanket to wrap the newborn. The newborn girl is eerily quiet and appears somewhat lethargic. As you confirm that the fire fighter and his partner, EMT fire fighter Steams, will maintain care of the mother, you quickly carry the infant inside the warm ambulance to perform an assessment.

Question 2

What is the best way to move the mother from the car to the back of the rig?

Once inside the warm ambulance with the neonate, you perform the APGAR and primary assessment (Table 1, Table 2). You also obtain a set of baseline vital signs (Table 3). Although you visualize chest rise and fall, the newborn still has yet to cry and you are feeling a bit anxious about it. Crying babies have a patent airway and are breathing. This newborn is too quiet.

Table 1 APGAR Score for Newborn at 1 minute

Appearance	1
Pulse	2
Grimace	0
Activity/muscle tone	1
Respiration	2
Total score	6

Table 2 Primary Assessment Findings for Newborn

General impression	Neonate girl, appears to be full-term.
Chief complaint	None.
Level of consciousness	Alert.
Airway	Open and patent.
Breathing	Lung sounds are clear and chest rise is equal bilaterally. Respiratory rate and effort are within normal limits.
Circulation	Rapid and strong brachial pulse is present. No external bleeding is noted. Skin is cool, dry, and pink in the core, with slight cyanosis noted to the fingers and toes.
Life threats	None.
Pain	Unknown.
Pertinent Negatives	None.
Pupils	Not obtained.
Glasgow coma scale (GCS)	Score: 12 (eye opening, 4; verbal response, 2; motor response, 6).
Interventions	Dry and warm neonate. Suction with bulb syringe. Blow-by oxygen administered.

Table 3 Baseline Vital Signs for Newborn

Respirations	44 breaths/min and regular
Pulse	150 beats/min and regular
Skin	Core warm. Extremities are cool to the touch, but not cold
Blood pressure	N/A
Oxygen saturation	Did not obtain

Question 3

As you begin to assess this infant, what assessment tools can you use?

Question 4

What are your immediate thoughts about why this infant is not crying yet?

You continue to dry the infant off and wrap her more snugly in the blanket, then put a foil baby bunting around the blanket to retain heat. You provide oxygen via blow-by method with a pediatric nonrebreathing mask and gently rub her back a little until she begins to cry and her skin pinks up.

Meanwhile, the fire fighters and Marty have brought the mother to the back of the ambulance on the gurney, her husband by her side. She still looks dazed, but wants to know how their baby girl is doing. You set the infant in her arms and prepare to assess the APGAR for a second time Table 4.

Table 4   APGAR Score for Newborn at 5 minutes

Appearance	2
Pulse	2
Grimace	2
Activity/muscle tone	2
Respiration	2
Total score	10

You are relieved to see that the newborn's condition has improved and her APGAR score has increased.

You ask the mother what she is going to name the baby. She tells you the baby's name is Katherine Elizabeth. The mother goes on to tell you that this is her third child and that because the hospital is just a few miles from home she and her husband had waited until the last minute to leave.

Question 5

At this point during the call, with the infant stabilized, what questions should you ask the mother?

Now that Katherine is stable, warm, dry, and in her mother's arms, you ask the mom her name and begin to gather a SAMPLE history from her, including her signs and symptoms, allergies, medications, pertinent past medical history, last oral intake, and events leading up to the injury or illness Table 5. She tells you her name is Amy. Katherine was delivered at 39 weeks. She tells you this pregnancy, like her previous two, was uncomplicated. She has been seeking obstetric care for the duration of the pregnancy and had an ultrasound done at 28 weeks. You ask if she could possibly be carrying twins or multiples and she replies "No."

Table 5 SAMPLE History for Amy

Signs and symptoms	Multigravida woman gave birth.
Allergies	No known drug allergies.
Medications	Prenatal multivitamins.
Pertinent past medical history	Pregnancy.
Last oral intake	Dinner about 5 hours ago.
Events leading up to the illness or injury	Heading to hospital in labor when started to deliver baby in the front seat of the car.

As you finish obtaining a history from Amy, she tells you she feels contractions again and thinks the placenta is getting ready to deliver. You have Marty hold the newborn while Amy pushes out the placenta. You position yourself at the vaginal opening and prepare to deliver the placenta with a red bag in hand. After a few pushes, the placenta delivers normally. You quickly inspect the placenta for any tears and find nothing unusual, then put it in the red bag, and secure the bag shut for transport to the receiving hospital. You place a large sterile pad at the vaginal opening to help control bleeding. Katherine is then placed in Amy's arms and Amy chooses to begin breastfeeding. You also tell Amy that you will massage her abdomen before transport begins to further control any vaginal bleeding. You use this time to complete your primary assessment of Amy **Table 6**.

Table 6 Primary Assessment Findings for Amy

General impression	34-year-old woman just given birth to baby in front seat of personal vehicle.
Chief complaint	None.
Level of consciousness	Alert.
Airway	Open and patent.
Breathing	Lungs sounds are clear and chest rise is equal bilaterally. Respiratory rate and effort are within normal limits.
Circulation	Strong and regular radial pulse is present. Some vaginal bleeding noted. Skin is warm, dry, and pink.
Life threats	None.
Pain	Some abdominal pain, 4 on a scale of 1 to 10.
Pertinent negatives	No difficulty breathing. No vaginal tearing.
Pupils	Pupils are equal, round, regular in size, and react properly to light (PEARRL).
Glasgow coma scale (GCS)	Score: 15 (eye opening, 4; verbal response, 5; motor response, 6).
Interventions	Passive warming with blankets. Fundal massage. Bleeding control.

Question 6

What are the transport considerations for the mother and newborn?

With both mother and newborn stabilized and resting comfortably, you tell Marty to begin heading toward Strong Memorial Hospital. Amy's husband says he will follow behind in his car and meet you at the hospital. Fortunately, it is only a short drive to the emergency department (ED). Marty has notified the ED that you will be arriving soon with a newborn and mother.

En route to Strong Memorial Hospital, you complete a full set of vital signs for Amy and a second set of vital signs for Katherine Table 7, Table 8.

Table 7 Baseline Vital Signs for Amy

Respirations	26 breaths/min and regular
Pulse	120 beats/min and regular
Skin	Pink, warm, and dry
Blood pressure	128/88 mm Hg
Oxygen saturation	98% on room air

Table 8 Second Set of Vital Signs for Katherine

Respirations	48 breaths/min and regular
Pulse	148 beats/min and regular
Skin	Extremities and body are warm and pink
Blood pressure	N/A
Oxygen saturation	98% on room air

The obstetrics (OB) staff and neonatal team from the 4th floor is awaiting your arrival at the ED entrance. They escort you to the elevator and the crew, patients, and father ride up to the labor and delivery floor. Dr. Tricia Clasgens is the OB attending. She begins talking with Amy and takes a quick look at Katherine, who is resting quietly in Amy's arms. Once up on the labor and delivery floor, the nurses help Amy over to a hospital bed and place the baby on an infant warming bed to assess her length and weight. At this point, Dr. Clasgens turns to you and asks "What was the time of delivery?" You look up with a surprised look on your face. With all the commotion of the delivery in the cold, you had not really noticed the time. Pulling out your pager, you look for the time of call and give this to Dr. Clasgens, who agrees this is probably as close to the actual time as you can get for time of delivery. Care is transferred over to the labor and delivery staff. You say your congratulations to Amy and her husband and leave to complete your paperwork and clean up the rig.

Question 7

What documentation considerations do you now have for this call?

Case Analysis

■ Question 1

What questions would you ask during your primary assessment on this patient? What concerns do you have for the mother and newborn?

The first point to note is that you have two patients on this call, the mother and baby. Question the attending EMT fire fighter carefully in regards to the delivery. Was the baby already delivered prior to his arrival? Is the mother stable? Are there any complications such as vaginal hemorrhage or umbilical prolapse? How does the infant appear? Does the mother or baby require immediate lifesaving interventions? Remember that the infant was just delivered in an unstable environment. Immediately move the infant to the ambulance and manage the airway. The weather conditions make this call a challenge until both patients are safe inside the heated ambulance.

■ Question 2

What is the best way to move the mother from the car to the back of the rig?

While you attend to the needs of the infant, the EMT fire fighter will need to maintain patient control of the mother. Caution should be used in transferring the mother to the back of the ambulance. Advise the attending fire fighter that the mother should not be allowed to walk or stand but, rather, should be lifted out of the vehicle to the gurney. Immediately after delivery, there is a risk that the mother may have a syncopal episode or exaggerate any existing bleeding.

■ Question 3

As you begin to assess this infant, what assessment tools can you use?

One assessment "tool" that you have to use is the pediatric assessment triangle (PAT) Figure 1 . This is a helpful tool to use to begin your assessment of any infant or child. The PAT is used in conjunction with your regular patient assessment. It consists of assessing appearance, work of breathing, and circulation to the skin.

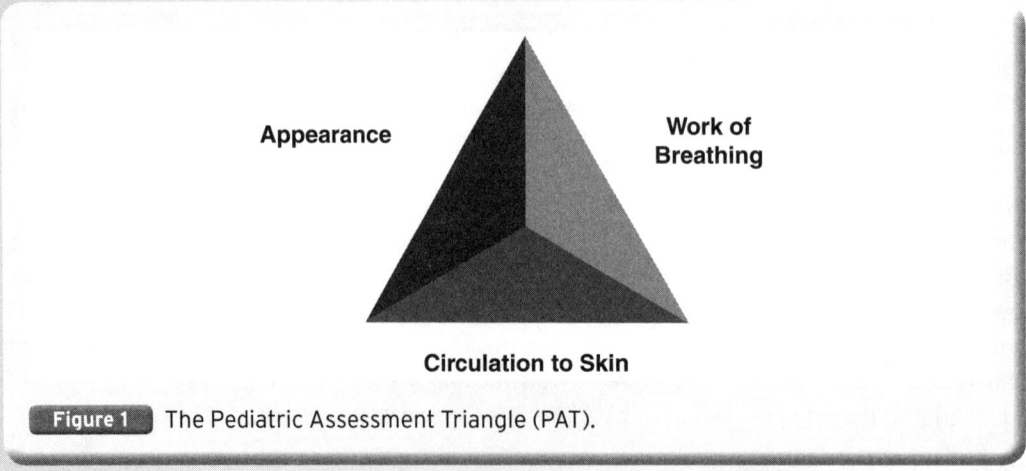

Figure 1 The Pediatric Assessment Triangle (PAT).

In addition, you should perform an APGAR assessment on this neonate **Table 9**. The APGAR score is a standard scoring system used to assess the status of a newborn, in both prehospital and hospital settings. The system works by assigning a numeric value (0, 1, or 2) to five areas of activity of the newborn baby.

Table 9 APGAR Scoring System

Area of Activity	Score 2	Score 1	Score 0
Appearance	Entire infant is pink.	Body is pink, but hands and feet remain blue.	Entire infant is blue or pale.
Pulse	More than 100 beats/min.	Fewer than 100 beats/min.	Absent pulse.
Grimace or irritability	Infant cries and tries to move foot away from finger snapped against sole of foot.	Infant gives a weak cry in response to stimulus.	Infant does not cry or react to stimulus.
Activity or muscle tone	Infant resists attempts to straighten hips and knees.	Infant makes weak attempts to resist straightening.	Infant is completely limp, with no muscle tone.
Respiration	Rapid respirations.	Slow respirations.	Absent respirations.

The first area of activity that is assessed is appearance. Shortly after birth, the skin of a light-skinned newborn and the mucous membranes of a dark-skinned infant should turn pink. It is not uncommon for newborns to have cyanosis of the extremities for a few minutes after birth, but the hands and feet should "pink up" rather quickly. Blue-colored skin or mucous membranes signal central cyanosis, which may be an indication of poor perfusion or poor circulatory function.

Pulse is the next step in assessing the APGAR score. Measuring pulse rates in newborns can be done using either a stethoscope or feeling for a brachial pulse or a pulse in the umbilical cord. As with any other patient without a pulse, the pulseless newborn will require immediate CPR.

Grimace or irritability is assessed by checking for crying or a withdrawing response to stimuli. One way to test for this is to snap your finger against the sole of the newborn's foot. A normal reaction from the newborn would be to pull the foot away, cry, or grimace to the stimuli.

Next in the APGAR assessment is to check for activity or muscle tone. The degree of muscle tone indicates oxygenation of the newborn's tissues. Normally, the hips and knees are flexed at birth, and, to some degree, the infant will resist attempts to straighten them out. A newborn should not be floppy or limp.

Last on the APGAR scoring system is to assess respiratory status and effort. In a healthy newborn, respirations will be rapid and regular, with a good, strong cry. If the respirations are slow, shallow, or labored, or if the cry is weak or absent, the newborn may be having respiratory difficulties and will need ventilatory assistance.

A perfect score on the APGAR scale is 10. Not all newborns will score 10 on the first assessment. The APGAR score should be calculated at 1 minute after birth and then again at 5 minutes after birth. Most newborns score between 7 and 8 at 1 minute and score 8 to 10 on the second evaluation.

■ Question 4

What are your immediate thoughts about why this infant is not crying yet?

This infant is most likely cold. Newborns are used to a warm environment in the womb of 98.6°F (37.4°C). Being in a cold environment diminishes a newborn's responses and reflexes. Newborns and infants are not able to compensate well for temperature changes because their thermoregulatory systems are immature. In addition, this infant may need airway suctioning, physical stimulation, and oxygen support.

If meconium (fetal stool) was present at birth, the first bowel movement might have inadvertently entered the newborn's airway. If this is the case, aggressive suctioning is necessary to remove as much meconium as possible from the newborn's airway. Viscous (thick secretions) meconium can impede the infant's airway, leading to respiratory distress or full airway obstruction. Vigorous suctioning of the infant's mouth and oropharynx prior to the body being delivered may help prevent meconium from being inhaled into the airway.

■ Question 5

At this point during the call, with the infant stabilized, what questions should you ask the mother?

Questions to ask include:
- How many pregnancies have you had?
- How many live births have you had?
- When was your due date?
- Did you have any complications during this pregnancy?
- Were you under the care of an obstetrician or other physician during this pregnancy?
- Do you have a history of diabetes?
- Do you have any bleeding disorders?
- Was this a high-risk pregnancy?
- Could you be expecting multiples?
- Do you have any medical conditions?
- Do you take any medications?
- When was the last time you ate?
- When did the contractions start?
- When did you feel the urge to push?
- Have you experienced post-delivery complications in previous pregnancies?
- Are you experiencing any dizziness, lightheadedness, or nausea?
- Are you experiencing any abnormal pain?
- Do you feel the urge to push again?
- Have you delivered the placenta?
- Are you experiencing any contractions right now?
- How did your previous deliveries progress?

Question 6

What are the transport considerations for the mother and newborn?

The mother should be transported on the gurney with lap belts and shoulder belts fastened in place. There is much controversy about how newborns should be transported. In the past, infants born in the prehospital setting have been carried in the arms of their mothers, who are generally seated on the gurneys, or stretchers, in the ambulance. While there are some benefits to both the mother and her baby in this situation (such as the mother's body temperature keeping the baby warm and the ability to breastfeed), this traditional practice of transport has come under scrutiny in recent years. Just as infants are not safe riding on the laps of passengers in personal vehicles, they are also not safe riding unrestrained in the back of ambulances. Each agency should review what strategies they will use when faced with this unique situation in prehospital care.

Question 7

What documentation considerations do you now have for this call?

Now that you have two patients, you will have two PCRs! Be sure to include the following in your documentation:

Documentation Tips for the Mother	Documentation Tips for the Infant
• Date, time, and location of birth	• Date, time, and location of birth
• Time of delivery for the placenta	• Initial and secondary APGAR scores for the infant
• What the placenta looked like (any tears?)	• General appearance of the infant after birth and during transport
• Any excessive bleeding?	
• The number of pads needed to control the vaginal bleeding	• Any presence of meconium?
• Whether the mother breast fed or not	• If suctioning was needed to clear the airway
• Was fundal massage used?	• Was resuscitation needed of the infant?
• Any tearing noted to the vagina after birth?	• When the umbilical cord was cut and clamped (and by whom?)
• Any complications during the birth?	• Any abnormalities noted to the umbilical cord or placenta?
• Was there any bleeding prior to the birth?	
• Patient history	• Any abnormal findings in the infant?
• Any assessments or treatments performed on the mother?	• Any treatments performed on the infant?
• Method of transport	• Method of transport

Patient Care Report for Amy

EMS Patient Care Report (PCR)

Date: 01-18-2008	Incident No.: 0122	Nature of Call: Childbirth		Location: 2200 Hiawatha Avenue	
Dispatched: 2332	En Route: 2333	At Scene: 2336	Transport: 2352	At Hospital: 0005	In Service: 0045

Patient Information

Age: 34 years	**Allergies:** None
Sex: Female	**Medications:** Prenatal multivitamins
Weight (in kg [lb]): 75 kg (166 lb)	**Past Medical History:** Pregnancy
	Chief Complaint: None

Vital Signs

Time: 2355	BP: 128/88	Pulse: 120 and regular	Respirations: 26 and regular	SpO$_2$: 98% on ambient air
Time:	BP:	Pulse:	Respirations:	SpO$_2$:
Time:	BP:	Pulse:	Respirations:	SpO$_2$:

EMS Treatment
(circle all that apply)

Oxygen @ <u>15</u> L/min via (circle one): NC NRM Bag-mask device Blow-by	Assisted Ventilation	Airway Adjunct	CPR
Defibrillation	**(Bleeding Control)**	Bandaging	Splinting	**(Other:)** Assited with delivery of the placenta; fundal massage; passive warming

Narrative

Ambulance 3059 was dispatched to a parking lot for a woman in labor. Upon arrival to the scene, neonate found in the arms of EMT fire fighter Preston, cord still attached. EMT fire fighter Preston was holding the newborn while suctioning her airway. EMT fire fighters Preston and Stearns then clamped and cut the cord. Medic took baby in large blankets to the warmth of the ambulance for evaluation. Mother said she and her husband were on their way to Strong Memorial Hospital for delivery of their third baby when she had the urge to push. Her husband pulled the car over in the parking lot of the coffee shop and went inside to make a phone call to 9-1-1. When the father came back outside, his wife had just delivered the baby girl on the floor of the front seat of the car. Fire first response arrived just after the baby was delivered and began care of the infant. Mother stated she has had 2 previous pregnancies that all ended in live births. She stated she was 39 weeks pregnant with this baby and had been seeking obstetric care throughout her healthy pregnancy. Once the cord was clamped and cut, infant given to medic to carry to ambulance in blanket. Delivery of the placenta occurred approximately 12 minutes after our arrival on scene and was without complications or excessive bleeding. Obstetrics pads were used at the vaginal opening to control bleeding and fundal massage was performed en route to the hospital. Obstetrics pad needed to be replaced just once en route to the hospital. After fundal massage for about 10 minutes, vaginal bleeding slowed. Both mother and infant remained stable en route to the hospital. Medical personnel from the labor and delivery floor greeted us at the ED entrance and escorted us up on the elevator to the 4th floor. Reports on mother and baby were given to Dr. Clasgens and care was transferred over to the labor and delivery staff in room 4231. **End of report**

Patient Care Report for Katherine

EMS Patient Care Report (PCR)

Date: 01-18-2008	Incident No.: 0123	Nature of Call: Childbirth	Location: 2200 Hiawatha Avenue
Dispatched: 2332	En Route: 2333	At Scene: 2336	Transport: 2352	At Hospital: 0005	In Service: 0020

Patient Information

Age: 1 hour
Sex: Female
Weight (in kg [lb]): 3.5kg (7 lb)

Allergies: No known allergies
Medications: None
Past Medical History: None
Chief Complaint: None

Vital Signs

Time	BP	Pulse	Respirations	SpO$_2$
2346	Not obtained	150 and regular	44 and regular	Not assessed
2355	Not obtained	148 and regular	48 and regular	98% on room air

EMS Treatment (circle all that apply)

Oxygen @ **15** L/min via (circle one): NC NRM Bag-mask device **(Blow-by)**	Assisted Ventilation	Airway Adjunct	CPR
Defibrillation	Bleeding Control	Bandaging	Splinting	**(Other:)** Dried and warmed infant

Narrative

Ambulance 3059 was dispatched to a parking lot for a woman in labor. Upon arrival to the scene, neonate found in the arms of EMT fire fighter Preston, cord still attached. EMT fire fighter Preston was holding the newborn while suctioning her airway. EMT fire fighters Preston and Stearns then clamped and cut the cord. Medic took baby in large blankets to the warmth of the ambulance for evaluation. Mother said she and her husband were on their way to Strong Memorial Hospital for delivery of their third baby when she had the urge to push. Her husband pulled the car over in the parking lot of the coffee shop and went inside to make a phone call to 9-1-1. When the father came back outside, his wife had just delivered the baby girl on the floor of the front seat of the car. Fire first response arrived just after the baby was delivered and began care of the infant. Mother stated she has had 2 previous pregnancies that all ended in live births. She stated she was 39 weeks pregnant with this baby and had been seeking obstetric care throughout her healthy pregnancy. Once the cord was clamped and cut, infant given to medic to carry to ambulance in blanket. Infant was immediately warmed by completely drying infant and using blankets to swaddle. Assessment of infant revealed: HR of 150, respiratory rate of 44 and regular, brachial pulses were strong. Core of infant was initially warm with cool extremities. First APGAR score was 6 (A, 1; P, 2; G, 0; A, 1; R, 2). Upon assessing the infant's airway, no fluids were visible, breathing was not noisy, and chest expansion was equal bilaterally; brachial pulses remained strong throughout transport. Once the infant was warmed up, she began to cry. APGAR was then reevaluated at approximately 5 minutes and was a 10. Infant was monitored and kept warm en route to the hospital. Medical personnel from the labor and delivery floor greeted us at the ED entrance and escorted us up on the elevator to the 4th floor. Reports on mother and baby were given to Dr. Clasgens and care was transferred over to the labor and delivery staff in room 4231. **End of report**

CASE STUDY 24

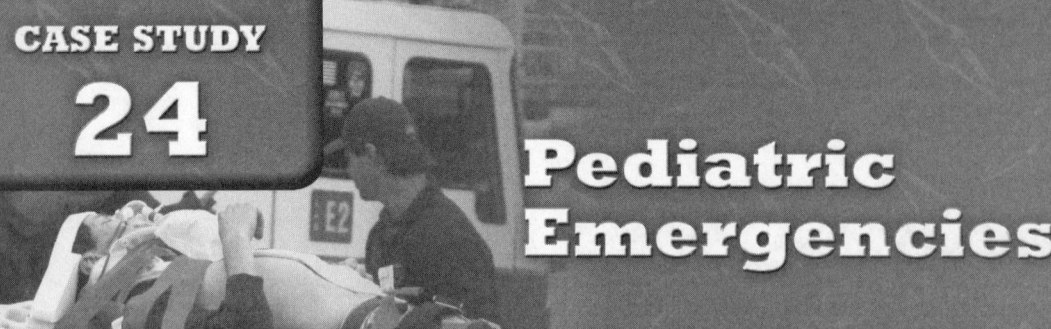

Pediatric Emergencies

Girl With Cold-Like Symptoms

It is the first of July. You have just finished transferring care of your patient to the emergency department (ED) staff at one of your local hospitals and you are preparing to leave when your partner, Lamar, tells you there is another call for service in your district and asks if you are ready to take it. You let Lamar know your patient transfer is complete and that you are ready to take the next call. You and Lamar head for the address given by dispatch. Dispatch advises that the call is for a 5-year-old girl with a cold at 2578 Fullmont Drive. Time out is 2133 hours.

You arrive on scene to find the patient in her mother's arms at the end of the driveway. The child's mother tells you her daughter's name is Makeda. The girl has no apparent physical injuries, and you expect this will be a quick call. As you move in closer, however, you notice Makeda is having difficulty breathing. You begin to suspect this is much more than a simple "cold."

As you begin to assess the scene, you realize that the mother does not speak much English; however, her older sister is present and offers to translate. The older sister introduces herself and tells you that the family recently moved to the United States from Ethiopia and that her mother's name is Faiza.

Question 1

What should you be concerned about at this scene?

As you are gathering a history of the present illness, you assist the mother and Makeda into the back of the ambulance for further assessment. Once in the ambulance, you ask Makeda what is bothering her. She says her stomach hurts, but otherwise makes no complaints and is quiet. Faiza is obviously concerned and is telling you that Makeda is not behaving normally.

Due to her breathing abnormality, you decide it would be best to transport Makeda as soon as possible to the nearest hospital. You ask Makeda's older sister, Selam, if she would be willing to ride along in the ambulance in case you need an interpreter. She agrees and is belted in the front passenger seat. After securing Makeda to the gurney and Faiza to the bench seat, you begin transport to Camden Children's Hospital, which is just 5 miles away.

During your primary assessment you found that Makeda has an open airway and will answer your questions when asked, but remains quiet. As you assess Makeda's breathing further, you noted nasal flaring with a rapid and shallow respiratory rate.

Question 2

Why do you think Makeda is having respiratory difficulties?

Question 3

What can be done to ease her respiratory difficulties?

You tell Makeda and her mother that you are going to give her some oxygen through a little mask. Makeda looks at you with some apprehension in her eyes. You tell her it is just some air that will help her to breathe better. She complies with the nonrebreathing oxygen mask, which you have set at 15 L/min. After ensuring that Makeda's airway and breathing have been assessed and treated, you offer her a small stuffed elephant to hold in the hopes that this will bring her some comfort for the remainder of the evaluation and transport to the hospital. She takes it eagerly and hugs it tightly.

You use this opportunity to assess her circulation to complete her primary assessment **Table 1**. She has strong, rapid radial pulses. There is no bleeding anywhere on her body that you can see. Her skin is warm and dry, and the mucosa in her eyes is pink.

Table 1 Primary Assessment Findings for Makeda

General impression	5-year-old girl with stomach ache.
Chief complaint	Stomach pain.
Level of consciousness	Alert to people and surroundings.
Airway	Patent airway with no apparent obstructions.
Breathing	Rapid shallow respirations.
	No apparent trauma.
Circulation	Strong, rapid radial pulse.
	No bleeding.
	Skin warm and dry and mucosa of eyes is pink.
Life threats	Possible breathing difficulties.
Pain	Stomach pain, unable to articulate severity.
Pertinent negatives	No trauma.
	No loss of consciousness.
	No nausea, vomiting, or diarrhea.
	No known exposure to toxins.
Pupils	Pupils are equal, round, regular in size, and react properly to light (PEARRL).
Glasgow coma scale (GCS)	Score: 15 (eye opening, 4; verbal response, 5; motor response, 6).
Interventions	Oxygen therapy via a nonrebreathing mask.

You then evaluate her vital signs Table 2, Table 3.

Table 2 — Normal Ranges for Pediatric Vital Signs

Age Range	Respirations (breaths/min)	Pulse (beats/min)	Systolic blood pressure (mm Hg)
Neonate (0 to 1 month)	30 to 60	90 to 180	50 to 70
Infant (1 month to 1 year)	25 to 50	100 to 160	70 to 95
Toddler (1 to 3 years)	20 to 30	90 to 150	80 to 100
Preschool age (3 to 6 years)	20 to 25	80 to 140	80 to 100
School age (6 to 12 years)	15 to 20	70 to 120	80 to 110
Adolescent (12 to 18 years)	12 to 20	60 to 100	90 to 110

Table 3 — Baseline Vital Signs for Makeda

Respirations	38 breaths/min and shallow with nasal flaring
Pulse	138 beats/min and regular
Skin	Warm and dry
Blood pressure	82/58 mm Hg
Oxygen saturation	94% on high-flow oxygen

Once Makeda's vital signs have been evaluated, you reassess her breathing by listening to her lung sounds. She has expiratory wheezing and continues with nasal flaring despite oxygen therapy. You talk to her calmly and try to coach her breathing to a slower pace. This seems to help, so you decide to reassess her vital signs Table 4.

Table 4 — Secondary Vital Signs for Makeda

Respirations	30 breaths/min and regular with decreased nasal flaring
Pulse	130 beats/min and regular
Skin	Warm and dry
Blood pressure	84/58 mm Hg
Oxygen saturation	98% on high-flow oxygen

Faiza is relieved to see her daughter doing better. She expresses to you that she was very worried when Makeda came in the house just before dinner not looking well. You ask her if there is any possibility that Makeda could have gotten in to any poisons or medications. She tells you she does not think so. She further explains to you, in broken English, that Makeda was outside playing in the yard with her brother for about an hour while she was making dinner for the family. When Makeda and her brother came in to the house to wash their hands for dinner, Makeda did not seem like herself. You ask more about what the mother noticed that was different about Makeda. She tries to explain that Makeda is usually very talkative and playful. When she came inside she was quiet and did not want to eat any of her dinner. That is when Faiza noticed Makeda seemed to have problems breathing and had her oldest daughter, Selam, call 9-1-1. You inquire again about the possibility of any type of poisoning. There are not many medications in the home and the ones they have are all "child proof." The family is not aware of any garden or lawn poisons as they do not use them. You obtain a SAMPLE history, including signs and symptoms, allergies, medications, pertinent past medical history, last oral intake, and events leading up to the injury or illness Table 5.

Table 5 SAMPLE History for Makeda

Signs and symptoms	Nasal flaring. Difficulty breathing. Stomach ache.
Allergies	No known drug allergies.
Medications	None.
Pertinent past medical history	None.
Last oral intake	At lunch time; toasted pita bread with hummus and lentils, and mango juice.
Events leading up to the injury or illness	Playing outside with her brother prior to dinner and the start of the signs and symptoms.

You arrive at the hospital and have your driver assist Faiza safely out of the back of the rig. Once you are rolling into the ED, you explain to Faiza that Makeda will be triaged first and then taken to a bed. There is no line for triage at the pediatric ED and you triage Makeda with Tina, a registered nurse. Once she has triaged Makeda, you transfer her to bed 2R. The registered nurse that will be caring for Makeda, Kevin, is with you when you transfer Makeda to her bed and leave the bed railings up and lower the bed. You give a brief history to Kevin and your assessment findings. As you wash your hands in the room, Kevin is preparing to give Makeda a nebulizer treatment to assist with her breathing. You say goodbye to Makeda and her family and wish them well.

Case Analysis

Question 1

What should you be concerned about at this scene?

Because it is evening and dark out at the time of the call, being aware of and concerned about your surroundings would be one scene consideration. Why does the family meet you at the end of the driveway and not in the house? Are there any animals in sight? Is this location on or near a busy road? If the parent does not speak English well, how will you communicate?

Question 2

Why do you think Makeda is having respiratory difficulties?

There are many reasons that Makeda could be having respiratory difficulties, including the following:

- Allergic reaction: Allergic reactions can be mild or severe, acute or chronic. Many allergies (seasonal, for example) affect the respiratory system. Food allergies affect approximately 6% of young children. The most common childhood food allergy is to milk, affecting 2.5% of children younger than 3 years; by age 16 years, 80% of children with this allergy have outgrown it.
- Asthma: According to the American Academy of Allergy, Asthma and Immunology, asthma rates in children younger than 5 years have increased more than 160% from 1980 to 1994. In 2005 alone, 8.9% of children in the United States currently had asthma. Nine million US children younger than 18 years have been diagnosed with asthma at some point in their lifetime. Nearly 4 million children have had an asthma attack in the previous year. As with adults, asthma causes airway narrowing and the production of mucus in the airways, making it difficult to breathe.
- Poisoning: Certain chemicals and over-the-counter and prescription medications can cause respiratory distress in children.
- Respiratory infections such as bronchiolitis, pneumonia, RSV (respiratory syncytial virus), croup, epiglottitis, and pertussis may result in respiratory distress in children.
- Bronchiolitis is a viral infection affecting infants (usually at 2 to 6 months, but up to age 2 years) that causes edema and mucus production in the lower, smaller airways. This often occurs in the winter months and follows an upper respiratory tract infection.
- Pneumonia can be viral or bacterial. It affects the lower airway and alveoli, making it difficult for gas exchange to take place.
- RSV is the most common cause of bronchiolitis and pneumonia among infants (birth to 1 year of age).
- Croup is a viral infection of the upper airway (larynx, trachea, and bronchi). Like asthma, it causes airway narrowing. Croup usually affects the area of the cricoid ring and is most prevalent during the fall and winter seasons. Children afflicted with croup have a characteristic "seal bark" cough.
- Epiglottitis is a bacterial infection of the epiglottis. This infection causes swelling of the epiglottis and can run the risk of complete airway obstruction.
- Pertussis is also known as whooping cough. This bacterial infection is highly contagious. Pertussis is known for its characteristic severe, hacking cough that sounds like a "whoop." Pertussis is a preventable disease, and many children in the United States have been immunized against it.

Question 3

What can be done to ease her respiratory difficulties?

Keeping your pediatric patient calm is a priority with any illness or traumatic injury. If your patient becomes more upset, this can make his or her condition worse. Administering high-flow oxygen and transporting Makeda in a position of comfort should help relieve some of her symptoms of respiratory distress.

Patient Care Report for Makeda

EMS Patient Care Report (PCR)						
Date: 07-01-2011		**Incident No.:**	**Nature of Call:** Difficulty breathing		**Location:** 2578 Fullmont Drive	
Dispatched: 2133	**En Route:** 2133		**At Scene:** 2139	**Transport:** 2151	**At Hospital:** 2202	**In Service:** 2221

Patient Information	
Age: 5 years	**Allergies:** No known allergies to medication
Sex: Female	**Medications:** None
Weight (in kg [lb]): 21.77 kg (48 lb)	**Past Medical History:** None
	Chief Complaint: Stomach ache

Vital Signs				
Time: 2144	**BP:** 82/58	**Pulse:** 138 and regular	**Respirations:** 38 and shallow	**SpO$_2$:** 94% on oxygen
Time: 2154	**BP:** 84/58	**Pulse:** 130 and regular	**Respirations:** 30 and regular	**SpO$_2$:** 98% on oxygen
Time:	**BP:**	**Pulse:**	**Respirations:**	**SpO$_2$:**

EMS Treatment (circle all that apply)				
Oxygen @ 15 L/min via (circle one): NC (NRM) Bag-mask Device		**Assisted Ventilation**	**Airway Adjunct**	**CPR**
Defibrillation	**Bleeding Control**	**Bandaging**	**Splinting**	**Other:**

Narrative

Responded to a single-family residence for a 5-year-old girl with stomach pain. On arrival family waiting outside for ambulance, with the patient being held in mother's arms. Mother explained that her daughter was outside playing with her brother before dinner. Mother said that patient is usually very talkative and energetic, but when patient came inside this evening, she was very quiet and not acting like herself. Patient moved to ambulance for assessment. Patient alert to her surroundings and people. Airway patent. Breathing is rapid and shallow and nasal flaring is present. Radial pulse is strong and rapid. There is no visible bleeding. Skin is warm and dry and mucosa is pink. Patient complains of stomach pain, but is unable to articulate on a pain scale. Family members confirm no trauma and no loss of consciousness. No known exposure to toxins and no recent nausea, vomiting, or diarrhea. PEARRL. GCS score of 15. Expiratory wheezes are heard during lung sounds assessment. Patient transported in position of comfort (sitting upright, seat belted on gurney). Due to close proximity of hospital, ALS was not called. Patient's older sister rode along in front compartment of ambulance (with seat belt) in case interpreter was needed as mother does not speak much English. Patient transported to Camden Children's Hospital and transferred to pediatric bed 2R. Left in the care of RN Kevin. Bed rails up and bed lowered. **End of report**

CASE STUDY 25

Geriatric Emergencies

Elderly Woman With Possible Hip Injury

You and your partner Taylor are driving back from Waterbury Hospital when a call comes in for an elderly woman who has fallen and has a possible hip injury. The location is 125 Johnsarbor Drive, South, Unit 215. The call is at a fairly new senior citizen housing complex about 3 miles from your location. You confirm the information with the dispatcher and turn the rig around to head in the direction of the call. Time out is 1038 hours.

Question 1

What can you infer from the dispatch information about this call?

You arrive at the secured facility and bring your equipment on the gurney to the front door. The security guard buzzes you in and directs you where to go. You take the elevator up to the second floor, get off, walk down the hall, and find unit 215 on the right. An employee of the housing complex greets you at the door and shows you into the small but well-kept and clean apartment.

Question 2

Why is it relevant to briefly inspect the surroundings of a patient's environment, especially that of an elderly patient?

You find your patient lying on the floor in the doorway of her bedroom. She is in the supine position and alert. You introduce yourself to her and ask her name. She tells you her name is Gertrude Sellman and then chuckles and says, "Please, call me Gertie." She begins to tell you what happened, and you can tell she has a patent airway. She also has good air exchange and does not seem to be having any difficulty breathing. You make a quick visual inspection around her and note there is no pooling of blood anywhere.

Gertie tells you she was walking from the living room into her bedroom when her shoe got caught on the carpeting and she fell in the doorway. She landed on her left side and hip. She tells you her hip hurts and she thinks she may have broken it.

Question 3

What type of consent are you obtaining from Gertie at this time?

You explain to Gertie that you need to assess her before you move her and ask if this is okay with her. She agrees and you continue with your primary assessment **Table 1** and obtain a set of baseline vital signs **Table 2**.

Table 1 — Primary Assessment Findings for Gertie

General impression	76-year-old woman, alert, lying supine on the floor due to an apparent fall.
Chief complaint	Left hip pain.
Level of consciousness	Alert and oriented to person, place, day, and event.
Airway	Intact and patent.
Breathing	Chest rise is equal bilaterally.
Circulation	Pulses strong and slightly irregular in both upper extremities.
Life threats	No apparent life threats. Need to rule out hip injury and need for transport to appropriate facility.
Pain	6 on a scale of 1 to 10.
Pertinent negatives	No apparent breathing difficulties or distress. Patient denies pain anywhere other than at injury site and denies loss of consciousness. No bleeding anywhere.
Pupils	Pupils are equal, round, regular in size, and react properly to light (PEARRL).
Glasgow coma scale (GCS)	Score: 15 (eye opening, 4; verbal response, 5; motor response, 6).
Interventions	Oxygen administration via a nonrebreathing mask.

Table 2 — Baseline Vital Signs for Gertie

Respirations	14 breaths/min and regular
Pulse	96 beats/min and slightly irregular
Skin	Warm, dry, and pink
Blood pressure	158/96 mm Hg
Oxygen saturation	99% on oxygen

Now that you have completed your primary assessment and obtained the patient's baseline vital signs, you assess Gertie's chief complaint, her left hip. You ask Gertie if anything hurts when you palpate her hips. She denies feeling any pain there and her pelvis feels intact. You then move your assessment down to her lower extremities. Gertie is wearing a skirt and you tell her you will need to take a quick look under her skirt to assess her thighs. She says she understands and you move her skirt up a bit to inspect both of her thighs. It is now apparent to you where Gertie's pain is coming from. There you see an obviously swollen and deformed left thigh, indicative of a femur fracture. You are surprised that Gertie is not crying out in pain as you understand femur fractures can be very painful. You do not find any swelling or deformity to the right side, and Gertie denies having any pain to the lower extremity on the right side.

Question 4

What is the best way to immobilize this injury?

Question 5

How will you proceed to move Gertie from the floor to the gurney?

After you explain to Gertie what you believe to be the source of her pain, you and your partner begin splinting her leg for a stable move to the gurney. While you splint, you obtain a SAMPLE history, including signs and symptoms, allergies, medications, pertinent past medical history, last oral intake, and events leading up to the injury or illness Table 3.

Table 3 Sample History for Gertie

Signs and symptoms	Visible swelling to left thigh.
Allergies	Shellfish and codeine.
Medications	Fosamax, Lotensin, Septra, Senekot, and multi-vitamin with iron.
Pertinent past medical history	Osteoporosis, hypertension, urinary tract infection (UTI).
Last oral intake	Breakfast this morning, including oatmeal, prune juice, coffee, and a danish.
Events leading up to the injury or illness	Tripped on carpeting and fell onto floor in apartment.

Once the traction device is on, along with a cold pack, Gertie feels some relief of pain. Because of Gertie's history of osteoporosis, you decide to move her from the floor to the gurney on a backboard, being careful to use a lot of padding on the board with blankets for her comfort.

Once inside the rig, you reassess Gertie's vital signs Table 4 and perform a secondary assessment Table 5.

Table 4 Second Set of Vital Signs for Gertie

Respirations	12 breaths/min and regular
Pulse	92 beats/min and slightly irregular
Skin	Warm, dry, and pink
Blood pressure	150/92 mm Hg
Oxygen saturation	100% on oxygen

Table 5	Secondary Assessment Findings for Gertie
Level of consciousness	Remains alert and oriented to person, place, day, and event. Talkative en route to the hospital.
Airway	Intact and patent.
Breathing	No apparent breathing difficulties or distress. Chest rise equal bilaterally.
Circulation	Pulses strong and slightly irregular in both upper extremities. No bleeding anywhere. Skin is warm, dry, and pink.
Head/neck	No DCAP-BTLS noted to head or neck. Patient denies head and neck pain.
Chest	Chest rise is equal bilaterally. Lung sounds clear bilaterally. No chest trauma. Patient denies chest pain or pressure.
Abdomen	Abdomen is soft, nontender, and without trauma.
Pelvis/genitalia	Pelvis is intact. No pain on palpation.
Lower extremities	Left thigh is swollen and deformed. Pulse, movement, and sensation are positive in both lower extremities. Patient has pain with all attempted range of motion of her lower extremities. No DCAP-BTLS noted to the lower right extremity.
Upper extremities	Upper extremities are positive for pulse, movement, and sensation. No DCAP-BTLS noted to upper extremities.
Back/neck	Back and neck are free from pain and DCAP-BTLS.
Pain	4 on a scale of 1 to 10.
Glasgow coma scale (GCS)	Score: 15 (eye opening, 4; verbal response, 5; motor response, 6).
Interventions	Traction splint secured to injured leg. Patient on backboard with padding for comfort and support. Oxygen therapy administered because of possible blood loss from fracture site. ALS not contacted because of proximity to hospital and a pain rating of 4/10 at time of transport.

You are close to Highland Hospital (where they specialize in geriatric care) and arrive in less than 15 minutes. After speaking with the triage nurse, you move Gertie to bed 3 in the trauma bay. Bed rails are up and the bed is lowered to the lowest position for safety. Patient care technician Peter Bradley is in attendance. You wish Gertie well and head out to wash up, clean up, restock, and complete your paperwork.

As you return to get some water after you have cleaned up the gurney and rig, one of the emergency care physicians calls you over to view Gertie's radiograph. She indeed has a midshaft femur fracture to the left leg.

Case Analysis

■ Question 1

What can you infer from the dispatch information about this call?

On the basis of the dispatch information, you can infer that this patient most likely resides at the senior citizen housing. If the patient has fallen with a possible hip injury, she probably will not be able to get up on her own. She may have had a call button that she used to contact 9-1-1.

■ Question 2

Why is it relevant to briefly inspect the surroundings of a patient's environment, especially that of an elderly patient?

Inspecting the environment of geriatric patients is the "E" in the GEMS diamond **Figure 1**. When you respond to calls for elderly patients, it is helpful to observe their surroundings to look for any potential hazards. EMS personnel may be the first to offer advice on safer living at an elderly patient's home. For example, if there are throw or scatter rugs spread about the floors, this would be noted as a potential tripping hazard. When you point out these potential hazards, the patient may be able to change the environment and prevent injuries.

G Geriatric Patients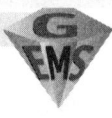
- Present atypically
- Deserve respect
- Experience normal changes with age

E Environmental Assessment
- Check for hazardous conditions that may be present (eg, poor wiring, rotted floors, unventilated gas heaters, broken window glass, clutter that prevents adequate egress).
- Are smoke detectors present and working?
- Is the home too hot or too cold?
- Is there an odor of feces or urine in the home? Is bedding soiled or urine-soaked?
- Is food present in the home? Is it adequate and unspoiled?
- Are liquor bottles present? If so, are they lying empty?
- If the patient has a disability, are appropriate assistive devices (eg, ramps, rails, wheelchairs, or walkers) present?
- Does the patient have access to a telephone?
- Are medications out of date or unmarked, or are prescriptions for the same or similar medications from many physicians? Are any of the medications prescribed to other people?
- If living with others, is the patient confined to one part of the home?
- If the patient is residing in a nursing facility, does the care appear to be adequate to meet the patient's needs?

M Medical Assessment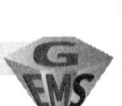
- Older patients tend to have a variety of medical problems, making assessment more complex. Keep this in mind in all cases—both trauma and medical. A trauma patient may have an underlying medical condition that could have caused or may be exacerbated by the injury.
- Obtaining a medical history is important in older patients, regardless of the chief complaint.
- Primary assessment
- Reassessment

S Social Assessment
- Assess activities of daily living (eating, dressing, bathing, toileting).
- Are these activities being provided for the patient? If so, by whom?
- Are there delays in obtaining food, medication, or other necessary items? The patient may complain of this, or the environment may suggest this.
- If in an institutional setting, is the patient able to feed himself or herself? If not, is food still sitting on the food tray? Has the patient been lying in his or her own urine or feces for prolonged periods?
- Does the patient have a social network? Does the patient have a mechanism to interact socially with others on a daily basis?

Figure 1 The GEMS diamond provides a concise way to remember the important issues of older patients.

Question 3

What type of consent are you obtaining from Gertie at this time?

The consent obtained from Gertie is informed consent. Gertie responds verbally in agreement to treatment, which is referred to as expressed or actual consent.

Question 4

What is the best way to immobilize this injury?

A traction device may be used for any midshaft femur fractures that do not have accompanying knee or ankle injuries. In some patients, however, especially geriatric patients, it may be too painful to pull traction on their injured extremity to apply a traction splint. If that is the case, securing the legs together, with a pillow or blanket between the legs, may be more suitable and less painful in this population. The goal is to immobilize the injured leg and do so as painlessly as possible for your patient.

Question 5

How will you proceed to move Gertie from the floor to the gurney?

There are a few options for moving your patient from the floor to the gurney. One way is using a backboard. The problem this presents is the need to roll the patient to one side. With some patients, rolling them can be very painful, even if it is to their "good," or uninjured, side. Oftentimes elderly patients will also have curvature to the spine, called kyphosis and spondylosis. Kyphosis is a forward curvature of the back caused by abnormal increase in the curvature of the spine. Kyphosis is sometimes referred to as "humpback" since the back curves outward. Spondylosis is a degeneration of the spine caused by wear and tear of the joints. Because the bones lose their formation, the patient's back or neck may appear curvy. Both of these spinal curvatures present a challenge to EMS providers because patients cannot lie down flat onto a backboard. Use special care when immobilizing a patient with one of these conditions. Extra padding is needed for comfort and security.

Another option for moving the patient is a scoop stretcher **Figure 2**. Scoop stretchers come apart into two pieces lengthwise. The advantage of the scoop stretcher is that you do not need to roll the patient. The stretcher comes apart and you place one side under the patient at a time. Once the pieces come together in the center of the patient, you secure the stretcher at the head and the foot with a latch system. The patient is then ready to be lifted, or scooped, off the ground or floor.

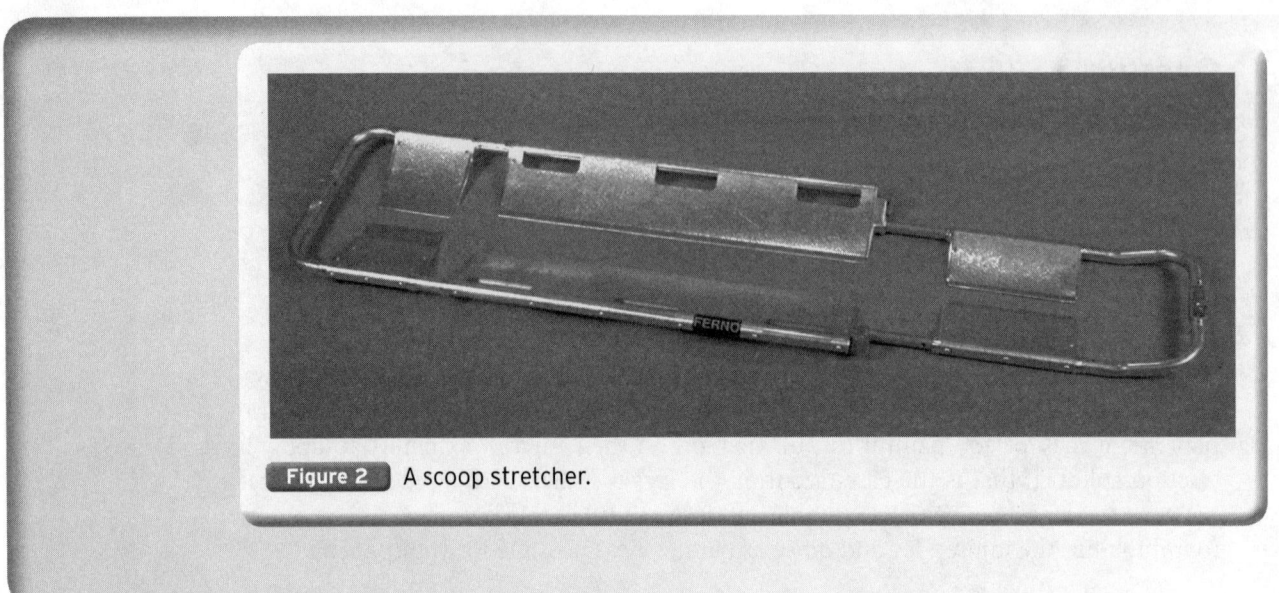

Figure 2 A scoop stretcher.

Patient Care Report for Gertie

EMS Patient Care Report (PCR)

Date: 06-25-2011	Incident No.: 354	Nature of Call: Fall		Location: 125 Johnsarbor Drive, South, Unit 215	
Dispatched: 1038	En Route: 1038	At Scene: 1046	Transport: 1111	At Hospital: 1127	In Service: 1150

Patient Information

Age: 76 years	**Allergies:** Shellfish and codeine
Sex: Female	**Medications:** Fosamax, Lotensin, Septra, Senekot, and multi-vitamin with iron
Weight (in kg [lb]): 60.78 kg (134 lb)	**Past Medical History:** Osteoporosis, hypertension, urinary tract infection (UTI)
	Chief Complaint: Left hip pain

Vital Signs

Time	BP	Pulse	Respirations	SpO$_2$
1049	158/96	96 and slightly irregular	14 and regular	99% on oxygen
1105	150/92	92 and slightly irregular	12 and regular	100% on oxygen

EMS Treatment (circle all that apply)

Oxygen @ 15 L/min via (circle one): NC (NRM) Bag-mask Device	Assisted Ventilation	Airway Adjunct	CPR
Defibrillation	**Bleeding Control**	**Bandaging**	**(Splinting)** Traction splint	**(Other:)** Cold pack

Narrative

Called to the residence of an elderly woman who has fallen. On arrival patient was found on the floor in the doorway of her bedroom. Patient is alert to crew. Patient states she fell when her shoe got caught on the carpet while walking to her bedroom. Patient denies losing consciousness and says she was able to call for help with her call button. Patient denies hitting her head. Patient states she fell onto her left side and hip. Patient aware of her surroundings, day, time, and event. Primary assessment reveals: patent airway, chest rise equal bilaterally with respirations, no shortness of breath or difficulty breathing; no visible signs of bleeding; strong and slightly irregular pulses present in upper extremities, skin warm, dry, and pink. Patient rates aching pain as a 6/10. PEARRL, GCS score of 15. Oxygen administered for possible internal bleeding. Further assessment of the injury site reveals that pelvis is intact but the left thigh is swollen and deformed in the midshaft area. Cold pack applied to injury site. Leg splinted with a traction device. Patient moved to backboard then to gurney. Remaining secondary assessment completed en route to ED. Secondary assessment findings are: patient remained alert and oriented for duration of transport; airway intact; breathing within normal limits and without complaints, lung sounds clear and chest rise equal bilaterally. Abdomen soft, nontender, and without trauma; pelvis intact and no pain on palpation; no DCAP-BTLS to lower right extremity; left lower extremity stabilized in traction splint and pulse, movement, sensation remain positive. Upper extremities were positive for pulse, movement, sensation and free of DCAP-BTLS; back and neck were also negative for DCAP-BTLS. Patient reported leg pain as 4/10 en route to hospital. GCS score remained 15. Patient triaged and moved to bed 3 in the trauma bay; bed rails up, bed lowered. Patient left in the care of patient care technician Peter Bradley. **End of report**

CASE STUDY 26

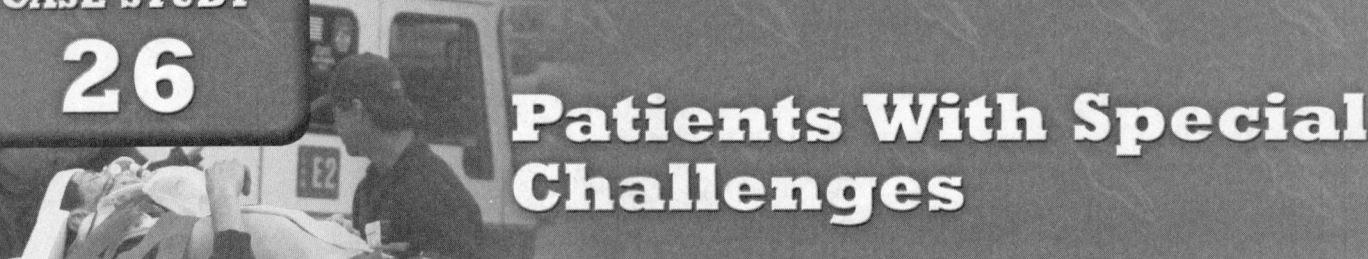

Patients With Special Challenges

Difficult Access to Hearing-Impaired Patient

On a pleasantly warm and sunny Wednesday evening in April, you and your driver, Laurie, receive a call for a 69-year-old woman who has fallen down a flight of stairs. The neighbor who called 9-1-1 stated that she cannot get into the front door because the patient is blocking the entrance. The address is 118 Larkspur Lane in the Quimbly Townhouse Complex. Time out is 1916. Since the caller indicated that she cannot gain access to the townhouse, the emergency medical services (EMS) dispatcher also called the fire department to assist with gaining entry to the home. ALS is en route to the call and is about twelve minutes out.

Upon arrival, you find the fire department on scene. Apparently the patient fell down a full flight of stairs that led to the front door. You and your partner, Laurie, as well as the fire fighters, wonder if you could gain access through the attached garage. When the garage door opens, everyone stands back in the driveway in amazement. The entire garage is packed with boxes and there is no way to even reach the door.

One of the fire fighters is able to pop the front window open, but the living room is also packed with large boxes. You can hear the patient calling out to you from the front entryway. "We'll be there as soon as we can. We're trying to get over to you now," you tell her, but you get no reply. The neighbor who called 9-1-1 comes over by the window to tell you the patient is hard of hearing and she may not be able to hear you if her hearing aid is not in. The neighbor also tells you your patient's name is Mrs. Ackerman. The fire fighters are now inside the home and are passing boxes out the window to make space to move around in the townhouse and get equipment and personnel in. There is literally no space inside the home.

Question 1

What safety concerns do you have for you and your crew? What safety concerns do you have for the patient?

Question 2

What strategies might you use to communicate with this patient if she cannot hear?

Once inside, you see stacks of magazines, dishes of pet food, pots and pans on the floor, and more boxes. The odor of cat urine permeates the air and stings your senses. At one point when you look up on top of the boxes you see cats. They are on boxes, under boxes, and on the floor. At first you see just three or four cats, but the further you venture inside, the more cats you see.

As you work your way over to the patient, you pull out a small notepad from your pocket and get your pen ready. Not knowing the degree of hearing loss, the pad of paper and pen may come in handy. As you get close to your patient, you wave your hand gently above her to get her attention and let her know you are there. You look directly at her and say "Hello." She looks up, relieved, and smiles and says "Hi." You ask her for her name and what exactly happened to her in an attempt to ascertain her level of consciousness. She gives you a quizzical look, indicating she did not understand you. After climbing over more boxes and rubble on the floor, you finally reach the patient. Now that you are kneeling near her side, you look directly at her again and ask her name. She tells you that her name is Mrs. Ackerman. Normally you would ask the patient where you could locate her hearing aid, but given her living conditions you don't think that is feasible. Fortunately, it seems like she has some lip reading ability. She tries to tell you that she was coming down the stairs when she tripped and fell down the entire staircase and landed on the floor. She says that her back and her neck hurt, but other than that she is okay. She thinks she fell almost two hours ago. The stairs that she fell down are littered with stacks of newspapers and magazines. Laurie takes head stabilization and you begin a primary assessment Table 1.

Table 1 Primary Assessment Findings for Mrs. Ackerman

General impression	69-year-old hearing-impaired woman who fell down a flight of stairs, awake and in pain.
Chief complaint	Back and neck pain.
Level of consciousness	Alert to person, place, day, and event.
Airway	Patent.
Breathing	Breathing is equal bilaterally.
Circulation	Skin is warm, pink, and dry.
	Radial pulses are strong and regular.
Life threats	Need to consider head and neck trauma due to the mechanism of injury (MOI).
Pain	Back pain rated as 6 on a scale of 1 to 10.
	Neck pain rated as 4 on a scale of 1 to 10.
Pertinent negatives	No trauma noted to the chest.
	No external bleeding is present.
Pupils	Pupils are equal, round, regular in size, and react properly to light (PEARRL).
Glasgow coma scale (GCS)	Score: 15 (eye opening, 4; verbal response, 5; motor response, 6).
Interventions	Spinal immobilization.
	Oxygen applied via nonrebreathing mask (NRM) due to MOI.

You obtain a SAMPLE history from Mrs. Ackerman, including signs and symptoms, allergies, medications, pertinent past medical history, last oral intake, and events leading up to the injury or illness. She cannot understand everything you are asking, so you write it down on your note pad Table 2.

Table 2 — SAMPLE History for Mrs. Ackerman

Signs and symptoms	Slight bruising noted to the right side forehead.
	Patient reporting pain to the neck and back.
Allergies	No known drug allergies.
Medications	Bentyl.
	Noncompliant with hypertension medications due to the side effects she experiences.
Pertinent past medical history	Irritable Bowel Syndrome (IBS).
	Hypertension.
Last oral intake	Unsure, probably sometime around lunch today.
Events leading up to the injury or illness	Coming down the stairs when she tripped and fell down the entire flight and landed on the floor.

You also have time to take a quick set of vital signs on Mrs. Ackerman while you wait for more personnel to assist with lifting **Table 3**.

Table 3 — Baseline Vital Signs for Mrs. Ackerman

Respirations	16 breaths/min and regular
Pulse	90 beats/min and irregular
Skin	Warm, dry, and pink
Blood pressure	160/90 mm Hg
Oxygen saturation	99% on oxygen

Question 3

What is significant about this patient having a history of hypertension and it not being controlled by medications?

Further history for Mrs. Ackerman reveals that she is widowed and lives alone with what looks to be at least a dozen cats. She denies any mental health problems and tells you she has a daughter in the area and a son who lives out of town. She is unsure of whether or not she lost consciousness after the fall. She is happy that her neighbor came to check on her as she was not able to get to a phone. You complete a secondary assessment **Table 4** and obtain a second set of vital signs **Table 5**.

Question 4

Are you concerned about the number of cats Mrs. Ackerman has and the condition in which she lives? If so, what are your concerns?

Table 4	Secondary Assessment Findings for Mrs. Ackerman
Level of consciousness	Alert and oriented to person, place, day, and event.
Airway	Intact and patent.
Breathing	Rate is within normal limits.
	No difficulty breathing.
	No pain upon inspiration.
	Lung sounds are clear and equal bilaterally.
	High-flow oxygen still administered via nonrebreathing mask.
Circulation	Pulses present in both upper extremities and remain strong and regular.
	Skin is warm, dry, and pink.
Head/neck	Bruise to right side of forehead.
	Pain to neck.
	No swelling noted upon palpation of neck.
	No other trauma noted to head or face.
	Pupils are sluggish bilaterally.
	Trachea is midline, no jugular vein distension noted.
Chest	No deformities, contusions, abrasions, punctures, penetrations, paradoxical motion in the chest, burns, tenderness, lacerations, or swelling (DCAP-BTLS) noted to chest.
	Lung sounds are clear and equal bilaterally with full expansion.
	Patient denies pain to chest or difficulty breathing.
Abdomen	Non-tender.
	No distention noted.
Pelvis/genitalia	Pelvis is intact with no deformities or pain on palpation.
	Patient denies any pain to the genitalia.
Lower extremities	No DCAP-BTLS noted to lower extremities.
	Pulse, movement, and sensation are present in both lower extremities.
Upper extremities	Swelling, deformity, and bruising are noted to right wrist.
	Pulse, movement, and sensation are present in left upper extremity.
	Sensation is present in right upper extremity, pulse is weak, and movement is difficult due to pain.
Back/neck	Patient reporting pain to the neck and upper back.
	Slight swelling noted to neck before application of cervical collar.
	Bruising noted to the upper back.
Pain	Neck pain 6 out of 10.
	Back pain 7 out of 10.
	Wrist pain 5 out of 10.
Glasgow coma scale (GCS)	Score: 15 (eye opening, 4; verbal response, 5; motor response, 6).

Patients With Special Challenges

Table 5	Second Set of Vital Signs for Mrs. Ackerman
Respirations	18 breaths/min and regular
Pulse	92 beats/min and irregular
Skin	Warm, dry, and pink
Blood pressure	156/86 mm Hg
Oxygen saturation	99% on oxygen

After the difficult task of extricating Mrs. Ackerman out of her disheveled home through the front window, the transport to Chandler Regional Hospital is rather uneventful. Mrs. Ackerman remains alert, oriented, and her vital signs remain stable. You call ahead to alert the emergency department (ED) to the need for a sign language interpreter, as you were unable to locate her hearing aids due to the cluttered conditions of the home. Upon arrival at the ED, there is a line at triage. Mrs. Ackerman asks if you will call her daughter to let her know what has happened.

Question 4

What specific information about Mrs. Ackerman's situation should you share with the triage nurse and why? Do you think it would be appropriate to speak to a social worker at the hospital on her behalf?

After speaking to the triage nurse, you move Mrs. Ackerman to a bed in the trauma bay. You ask Laurie if she will stay with Mrs. Ackerman while you speak to the nurse in private. You tell the nurse about the condition of Mrs. Ackerman's residence, including the hoarding of items and cats, and express your concern about her being discharged to her home in its current state. The nurse takes careful notes of what you say and puts it in a report. You know you will do the same on your patient care report. Before you leave to complete paperwork, the sign language interpreter walks in with Dr. Kresge by her side. You leave the bed rails up and lower the bed to its lowest position. You wish Mrs. Ackerman well and say goodbye.

Question 5

What are some unique findings from this call that would merit documentation?

Case Analysis

■ Question 1

What safety concerns do you have for you and your crew? What safety concerns do you have for the patient?

The safety concerns are evident from your scene size-up on this call. It appears Mrs. Ackerman is a "hoarder." Hoarding is often defined as the collecting of items, sometimes items that are considered worthless to others. People who have compulsive hoarding have an immense difficulty in discarding items and frequently have difficulty making decisions in life. Hoarding may also involve animals, which can create additional risk for the patient and the EMT.

Since you do not have access through the front door, you will need to choose another entry point. One safety concern for both patient and crew is stability in the scene. With clutter comes the potential to trip and fall.

Fire hazard is another serious risk when entering a hoarder's residence. The homes of hoarders pose an increased risk to the occupant, visitors, and rescue personnel. Excessive amounts of clutter in the residence make it very difficult not only to get to your patient, but also to retreat from the residence if the scene were to become unsafe. Because there is often a high volume of clutter, fires tend to burn faster and stronger. Additionally, there is an increased risk of fire damage to adjacent homes.

Research has been conducted on house fires where hoarding takes place and revealed that 25% of people who hoard do not believe they are hoarders; 77% are male and 73% are age 50 or older; fire incidents and fatalities occur across all metropolitan fire districts. Items that are commonly hoarded include:
- Magazines/newspapers/books
- Bills/receipts
- Clothing
- Greeting cards/letters
- Animals
- Pictures/photos
- Rubbish
- Records/tapes
- Collectibles
- Electrical appliances, equipment

■ Question 2

What strategies might you use to communicate with this patient if she cannot hear?

Although statistics vary according to the study, approximately 1 in 20 Americans is hard of hearing or deaf. This translates to roughly 10,000,000 hearing impaired people in this country. Of this number, less than 4% are under the age of 18.

It is normal to feel apprehensive when faced with a patient who has special needs or challenges. Communication with hearing impaired or deaf people may seem awkward initially, especially if you have never interacted with this population before. With patients who are hearing impaired, check to see if they have any assistive devices, such as hearing aids. If they do, see if they have them attached (usually behind or in the ear[s]) and on when you approach. If the hearing aids are nearby, such as sitting on the night stand, ask if they would like the hearing aids in. If a hearing impaired patient can hear better out of one ear over another, be sure to speak to that side of the patient so he or she has a better chance of hearing you.

Many hearing impaired and deaf people can read lips. In order for them to read your lips, however, they need to be able to see them. Do not hold your hands to your face or mouth when speaking to patients. Speak clearly and directly to the patient. If your patient is deaf and does not read lips, be sure to have pen and paper available to communicate. Currently, many cell phones have note-writing capabilities. Keep in mind that nonverbal communication is very important to deaf and hearing impaired people. Many times they get clues this way as to what you are trying to tell them. For example, you may have to gently touch a deaf or hard of hearing patient on the shoulder to get his or her attention. If you know sign language, use it. If you don't, consider learning a few common terms related to illness and injury in case you encounter a hearing impaired patient. Speak slowly and clearly, and make sure your position is good to a light source so the patient can see your lips and gestures as you speak. One other technique you can try with a hearing impaired patient is the "reverse stethoscope technique." This is where you put the earpieces of the stethoscope into the patient's ears, rather than your own, and speak into the diaphragm of the stethoscope to help amplify your voice.

■ Question 3

What is significant about this patient having a history of hypertension and it not being controlled by medications?

Patients with hypertension have a higher risk for cardiac events (such as heart attack and angina) and neurologic emergencies (such as stroke or transient ischemic attack [TIA]). Additionally, uncontrolled hypertension can lead to kidney damage, kidney failure, aneurysms, and dementia.

Patients can fall for a variety of reasons. Since uncontrolled hypertension can lead to strokes, for example, it is important to determine why the patient fell. A few questions to ask and assess on any call involving a patient who fell include:
- Did the patient fall because she tripped? If so, did she lose consciousness?
- Did she fall because she went unconscious?
- Did she fall because she had a heart attack?
- Did she fall because she had a stroke?
- Did she fall because she had a seizure?
- Did she fall because of drug or alcohol intoxication?
- Did she fall due to being hypoglycemic?

■ Question 4

Are you concerned about the number of cats Mrs. Ackerman has and the condition in which she lives? If so, what are your concerns?

Many people in America have pets in their homes. According to the Humane Society of the United States, there are approximately 77.5 million owned dogs and 93.6 million owned cats in the United States. Having more pets than one can care for should be a concern to providers entering a home. If the people living in the home are not caring for the animals properly, there is a high probability that they are also not caring for themselves properly. Over crowding of animals in homes can also lead to unsanitary conditions for both animals and people.

There are many different reasons why people hoard. For example, hoarders have emotional attachment to their belongings, and they believe their possessions are useful and therefore do not want to throw them away. Their belongings are reminders of people and events in their lives and discarding those belongings would resemble throwing out their memories. They may also hoard because it is too difficult of a task to organize and remove their possessions. In addition to the mentioned safety risks (fire hazards, egress concerns, etc.), hoarders are often socially isolated, too embarrassed to let others see how they live. This social isolation can have both physical and mental health ramifications. Living alone or socially isolated can lead to loneliness, depression, reduction in self care, increased risk of falls, and the inability to see health problems in oneself.

Question 5

What specific information about Mrs. Ackerman's situation should you share with the triage nurse and why? Do you think it would be appropriate to speak to a social worker at the hospital on her behalf?

As mentioned previously, there are many inherent safety risks in a hoarder's home. Since this tends to lead to social isolation, friends and relatives are often unaware of the severity of the situation. It would be important to alert the triage nurse and hospital staff of this situation so that social workers can get involved to offer mental health assistance to these patients. Many times EMS providers are the first people to see inside a person's home. As EMTs, we are in a unique position to observe a residence and make recommendations based on what is seen. We would be doing this patient a disservice if we did not speak up on her behalf and alert hospital personnel (such as doctors, nurses, and social workers) of her existing living arrangements. Being discharged back to the home of a hoarder is not safe.

Question 6

What are some unique findings from this call that would merit documentation?

Careful documentation is imperative on all calls. However, this type of call has some unique circumstances. One concern is the hoarding. As previously mentioned, hoarding can lead to social isolation, health and safety hazards, and depression. It is critical to document the patient's surroundings to paint a clear picture for the ED staff. Since her home presents a fire hazard and fall hazard, this information should be a consideration to them when they plan the patient's discharge. It would also be appropriate to document that the patient is deaf or hearing impaired. This would indicate the potential for some communication difficulties or need for additional resources. Some states have mandatory elder abuse reporting laws in effect. Although this does not appear to be an abusive situation, it could be helpful to contact elder services to inform them of her living conditions. It might be good to involve law enforcement in this instance, even though EMS providers are not necessarily mandated reporters (check with your state and local protocols), law enforcement could act as a conduit to services for the elderly and/or hoarding patient.

Patient Care Report for Mrs. Ackerman

EMS Patient Care Report (PCR)

Date: 04-16-2011	Incident No.: 654	Nature of Call: Person fallen		Location: 118 Larkspur Lane	
Dispatched: 1914	En Route: 1916	At Scene: 1927	Transport: 1948	At Hospital: 2002	In Service: 2030

Patient Information

Age: 69 years	**Allergies:** None
Sex: Female	**Medications:** Bentyl
Weight (in kg [lb]): 81 kg (180 lb)	**Past Medical History:** IBS, hypertension
	Chief Complaint: Back and neck pain

Vital Signs

Time	BP	Pulse	Respirations	SpO_2
1935	160/90	90 and regular	16 and regular	99% on oxygen
1950	156/86	92 and regular	18 and regular	99% on oxygen

EMS Treatment (circle all that apply)

Oxygen @ **15** L/min via (circle one): NC **(NRM)** Bag-mask device	Assisted Ventilation	Airway Adjunct	CPR
Defibrillation	Bleeding Control	Bandaging	**(Splinting:)** Splinted right wrist	**(Other:)** Cold therapy to right wrist at time of splinting due to swelling and pain; full spinal immobilization

Narrative

Called to the scene of a woman who had fallen and could not get up. Due to the difficulty gaining access to the residence, fire department was called to assist with entry. Unable to enter through the front door as the patient had fallen and landed in front of the door. Unable to gain access via the attached garage because there were too many boxes piled in the way of the door to the house. Access was finally gained by entering through a lower front window. Boxes in the residence needed to be moved out of the way so we could gain access to the patient. This took about five minutes to do before we could reach the patient. The neighbor informed us that our patient is hard of hearing. There is a strong odor of urine present in the home. When crew reached patient, communication was commenced using body language, writing on paper, and some lip reading. Patient told crew that she was coming down the stairs when she tripped and fell. Patient unsure if she lost consciousness or not. The stairs she fell down are a full flight and littered with magazines and other various items. Patient believed she may have fallen about two hours earlier. Patient's head was immediately stabilized and a primary assessment revealed: 69-year-old female who fell down stairs. Patient was alert and oriented and in pain. Her airway was patent and her breathing was unlabored. There was no visible trauma to her chest and breathing was equal bilaterally. Patient placed on high flow oxygen via NRM. Skin was warm, pink, and dry; no external bleeding present; radial pulses were strong and regular. Patient rated back pain as 6/10 and neck pain as 4/10. When obtaining a SAMPLE history, patient said she is not taking her hypertension medication currently because she "does not like the side effects." Patient was fully immobilized on long spine board and fire department assisted in moving patient out of house. Patient believed she last ate around lunchtime today. Patient also stated that she is a widow and lives alone. Patient denied any mental health history and said she has a daughter that lives in the area. Once patient was on board the ambulance, a secondary assessment was completed. Patient remained alert and oriented within normal limits for duration of transport. Airway also remained intact and unobstructed. Breathing rate was normal and patient denied any difficulty with breathing. No pain on inspiration. Lung sounds were clear and equal with expansion bilaterally. Strong pulses were present in both upper extremities. There was a bruise to the right side of her forehead. Pain in neck was now rated as 6/10. No swelling to neck and no other trauma noted to the face. Pupils were sluggish bilaterally. Trachea was midline and negative for jugular vein distention (JVD). No DCAP-BTLS to the chest. Abdomen was soft and nontender, no distention noted. Pelvis was intact with no deformities or pain on palpation. Patient denied any pain or injury to her genitalia. No DCAP-BTLS noted to lower extremities. Pulse, movement, and sensation were present in both lower extremities before and after immobilization to long spine board. Swelling, deformity, and bruising were noted to her right wrist. Wrist was immobilized with a padded splint and cold pack. Pulse, movement, and sensation were present in left upper extremity. Sensation was present in right upper extremity, pulse was weak, and movement was difficult due to pain. Patient reporting pain to the neck and upper back. Slight swelling noted to neck prior to application of cervical collar. Bruising noted to upper back but no deformities. GCS was 15. ALS transport to Chandler Regional Hospital was uneventful. Patient remained alert and oriented for duration of transport. Call placed to hospital to request sign language interpreter. Spoke to triage nurse, Maria, to alert her to the unsafe home environment that patient came from. Maria was made aware of the hoarding issue, which is a fire and safety hazard. Patient left in the care of Dr. Kresge and the sign language interpreter. Bed rails up, bed lowered, blanket left on patient. **End of report**

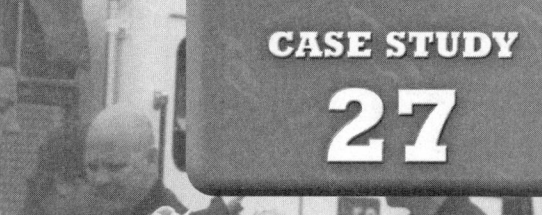

CASE STUDY 27

Lifting and Moving Patients

Girl Involved in Sledding Accident

It is a cold, sunny Saturday afternoon in March. The temperature is hovering around 32°F (0°C), when you and your partner, Yvonne, are called to Ellison Park for a sledding accident. The 9-1-1 dispatcher tells you that a 12-year-old girl struck a tree at the bottom of the hill while sledding with her family at a popular county park.

Once you arrive at the scene, you find a suitable location to park your ambulance. The area is crowded with parked cars and people sledding. The girl's father is anxiously awaiting your arrival at the top of the hill near the parking lot. He explains to you that they were enjoying the morning and had spent the past hour or so sledding, but the last time his daughter went down the hill she hit a tree. He ran down to check on her, and she tried to stand but couldn't put any pressure on her right leg, so he called 9-1-1. You glance down to where the girl's father is pointing. At the bottom of the hill, which looks to be about 30 yards away, in front of a pine tree, is the girl lying on the ground with her mother and sister by her side. The girl's father tells you she did not hit her head but did strike her right leg on the tree.

Question 1
What scene factors should you consider before heading down to your patient?

Question 2
What equipment should you and your partner take with you down the hill?

Question 3
What type of patient-moving device(s) might you consider using to move this patient safely from the bottom of the hill?

Prior to heading down to your patient, you call the fire department for lifting assistance, as you realize you will need help traversing back up the hill with the patient and gear. You also call for advanced life support (ALS) for pain management and possible fluid replacement. You get the medic bag, blankets, and splints from the ambulance, and Yvonne grabs the long board, straps, collars, and head blocks. Yvonne secures the equipment to the long board to make it easier to get down the hill while you ask the crowd to move away from the area where you will be going down to assess and retrieve the patient.

Yvonne has tied straps onto the front of the board and the foot of the board so you can lay the long board on the slope and guide it down, like a sled, holding onto the straps. You and your partner head down the hill carefully by side stepping and firmly planting your heels into the snow so you do not lose your balance. It is a slow and meticulous process, but you want to avoid falling. Once you finally reach the bottom, you can see that your patient, Clarissa, is alert to you and is talking to her mother. She also has a patent airway. You tell Clarissa and her family your name and let her know you are there to help. Her mother is very concerned that her right leg might be broken. You ask Clarissa to hold very still while Yvonne manually stabilizes her head and you begin your primary assessment **Table 1**.

Table 1 — Primary Assessment Findings for Clarissa

General impression	12-year-old girl injured in a sledding accident. Possible right leg injury.
Chief complaint	Pain to the lower right leg.
Level of consciousness	Alert and oriented to person, place, day, time, and event.
Airway	Patent.
Breathing	Breathing is unlabored. Chest expansion is equal bilaterally.
Circulation	Strong pulses present in both upper extremities. Skin is pale, cool, and dry.
Life threats	Long bone injury and potential internal bleeding.
Pain	8 on a scale of 1 to 10.
Pertinent negatives	No external bleeding. No trauma to the chest.
Pupils	Pupils are equal, round, regular in size, and react properly to light (PEARRL).
Glasgow coma scale (GCS)	Score: 15 (eye opening, 4; verbal response, 5; motor response, 6).
Interventions	Oxygen administered due to possible internal bleeding. Further assessment, treatment, and transport needed.

Question 4

Now that your primary assessment is complete, what would your next course of action be?

Because your patient has been lying in the cold snow for approximately 15 minutes, you choose to defer the vital signs assessment until you and your patient are in the warm environment of the heated ambulance. You would, however, like to perform a focused assessment of the leg injury prior to moving Clarissa. After covering your patient with blankets, you expose the injured leg to find it deformed and swollen. It is painful to the patient, even without palpation. The fire department has arrived and they have brought you a basket stretcher. You are happy to see them as you know you will need assistance getting your patient up the hill safely. One of the fire fighters now holds stabilization on your patient's injured leg. After removing Clarissa's boot, you complete a focused assessment **Table 2**.

Table 2: Focused Assessment for Clarissa

Pain	8 on a scale of 1 to 10.
DCAP-BTLS	Deformed and swollen lower right leg, tender to the touch.
	Negative for contusions, abrasions, punctures/penetrations, burns, and lacerations.
Circulation to the extremity	Negative for any external bleeding to injured leg.
	Posterior tibial pulse is present.
Motor function	Pulse, movement, and sensation are present in injured leg.
Sensory function	Movement and sensation are present in injured leg.

Another fire fighter helps you apply and secure appropriately sized padded splints. Pulse, movement, and sensation are reassessed and are still present. Once the cervical collar is applied, the fire personnel help you log roll Clarissa onto the backboard, while a fire fighter holds the immobilized leg. She is secured with straps, proper padding, and covered with the remaining blankets.

Question 5

What would be the safest way to get your patient to the top of the hill and to the ambulance?

The six fire fighters who brought the basket stretcher to you are ready to move your backboarded patient into the basket. Once in the basket, they secure her in place with the basket straps. You fasten the oxygen tank inside the basket stretcher to accompany your patient up the hill. An ALS provider has arrived at the top of the hill and tells you that he will set up in the back of the ambulance and wait for you there.

The fire fighters carry your patient up the hill with three people on each side of the basket stretcher. They move diagonally across the terrain while heading up the hill to the awaiting ambulance. You and Yvonne follow behind with the remaining equipment.

Once at the rear doors of the ambulance, the fire fighters put the basket stretcher down on the level ground, lift the backboard out, and place it on the awaiting gurney. Once in the warm ambulance, you assess baseline vital signs Table 3.

Table 3: Baseline Vital Signs for Clarissa

Respirations	24 breaths/min and regular
Pulse	116 beats/min and regular
Skin	Cool, pale, and dry
Blood pressure	100/68 mm Hg
Oxygen saturation	98% on oxygen

Andy, the paramedic, has given pain medication. Clarissa's dad will accompany you to the hospital, so Yvonne ensures that he is seated in the front passenger seat and is secured with a seat belt. You perform a secondary assessment and obtain a second set of vital signs en route to Children's Hospital of Wisconsin **Tables 4 and 5**.

Table 4 — Secondary Assessment Findings for Clarissa

Level of consciousness	Remains alert and oriented to person, place, day, time, and event.
Airway	Open and patent.
Breathing	Respirations within normal limits.
	Chest expansion is equal bilaterally.
	Lung sounds are clear.
Circulation	Radial pulses remain strong and regular.
	Carotid pulse is strong.
Head/neck	No pain to head or neck.
	Negative for DCAP-BTLS.
Chest	No chest trauma.
	Patient still denies any chest pain or pressure.
Abdomen	Soft, nontender, no pain on palpation.
Pelvis/genitalia	Pelvis is intact.
	Genitalia assessment deferred.
Lower extremities	Pulse, movement, and sensation are positive in both lower extremities.
	Right lower leg is swollen, distended, and painful.
	Left lower leg is without DCAP-BTLS and negative for pain.
Upper extremities	Upper extremities are negative for DCAP-BTLS.
	Pulse, movement, and sensation are positive.
Back/neck	No pain or deformities to back when assessed prior to boarding.
Life threats	Patient has an isolated long bone fracture to the lower right leg with possible internal bleeding.
Pain	Pain to lower right leg 3 on a scale of 1 to 10.
Pertinent negatives	Patient denies chest pain or pressure.
	Patient denies vomiting or losing consciousness.
	Parents confirm no loss of consciousness.
	Patient denies any pain to the head, neck, or back.
Pupils	Pupils are equal, round, regular in size, and react properly to light (PEARRL).
Glasgow coma scale (GCS)	Score: 15 (eye opening, 4; verbal response, 5; motor response, 6).
Interventions	Oxygen remains on high flow (15 L/min) via nonrebreathing mask (NRM).
	Injured leg splinted.
	Neurovascular function reassessed en route and without change.

Table 5 Second Set of Vital Signs for Clarissa

Respirations	22 breaths/min and regular
Pulse	100 beats/min and regular
Skin	Warm, pale, and dry
Blood pressure	100/66 mm Hg
Oxygen saturation	99% on oxygen

You are still a few miles from the hospital, so you take this time to obtain a SAMPLE history from Clarissa and her father, including signs and symptoms, allergies, medications, pertinent past medical history, last oral intake, and events leading up to the injury or illness **Table 6**.

Table 6 SAMPLE History for Clarissa

Signs and symptoms	Painful, swollen, and deformed lower right leg.
Allergies	None.
Medications	Children's multivitamin.
Pertinent past medical history	None.
Last oral intake	Lunch of soup and sandwich about 2 hours ago.
Events leading up to the injury or illness	Sledding down the hill when she struck a tree, legs first.

The remainder of your ride to the hospital is uneventful. You give a triage report to registered nurse (RN) Joleeta and move Clarissa to trauma bed 1. Side rails are left up and the bed is lowered. You leave Clarissa in the care of her father and emergency department (ED) staff.

Case Analysis

■ Question 1

What scene factors should you consider before heading down to your patient?

During your scene size-up, be sure to take into consideration the terrain where your patient is and where you will be heading. Additionally, you need to give forethought to the weather conditions. Is it raining, snowing, or windy? Are there extreme temperatures? Are there any animals (wildlife or domestic) that might interfere with access to your patient? Are there large crowds of people who may pose a threat to your safety? Are there any unstable surfaces you will be walking and working on? If so, how can you plan to move on those surfaces safely? Due to the ever-changing conditions and varying environments that EMS and fire personnel work in, it is imperative to dress appropriately for a call (including protective clothing, work boots, gloves, helmets, reflective vests, etc).

■ Question 2

What equipment should you and your partner take with you down the hill?

Now is the time to anticipate patient and equipment needs, before you head down the incline to your patient. Items to consider in this case:

- Personal protective equipment (PPE) such as gloves, goggles, face shields, and gowns
- Backboard with straps and head blocks
- Cervical collars
- Blankets
- Fully stocked medic bag with oxygen
- Splinting material
- Portable radios
- Automated external defibrillator (AED)

The equipment needed will depend on the illness or injury. Be prepared for the possibility of changes in condition, while only taking equipment that can be easily carried and transported back with the patient. If you determine that additional help will be needed, request it as soon as possible.

■ Question 3

What type of patient-moving device(s) might you consider using to move this patient safely from the bottom of the hill?

There are many types of patient-moving equipment available to use, all with unique features. The moving tool you use will most certainly depend on the location and situation in which your patient is found Table 7.

Table 7 Types of Patient-Moving Equipment

Patient Moving Device	When to Use
Stretcher or gurney	Rolls along the ground. Best used for smooth surfaces to transfer patients from the scene to the ambulance.
Backboard (long board)	Used to secure and move patients who must be immobilized due to potential spinal column injury. May be used to transfer patients from one surface or area to another.
Stair chair	Used to transfer conscious patients who have no traumatic injury to the spine up or down a flight of stairs.
Scoop stretcher	Generally used to "scoop" up a patient who may be in a difficult place to lift and move, who does not require spinal immobilization. For example, a patient with a possible hip fracture who is lying on the floor.
Basket stretcher	Shaped like a long basket, this can fit a backboard or scoop stretcher inside of it to assist moving a patient over rough terrain. Some basket stretchers are designed with holes in them to allow water or snow to drain from them. These basket stretchers are also used to lift people out of high-angle rescue situations, such as on the side of a mountain.
Flexible stretcher	This device can be rolled up for easy storage and is generally made up of canvas or synthetic material with carry straps.
Short backboard or vest-type device	Designed to immobilize patients whom you suspect of possible spinal cord injury. This device can be placed on the patient while in a seated position, such as in a car.
Blankets and sheets	Blankets can be used to transfer patients from one surface to another—for example, from a bed to a stretcher. They can also be used for an emergency move, such as the blanket drag, when a patient must be moved quickly to prevent further injury or death.

Question 4

Now that your primary assessment is complete, what would your next course of action be?

With your primary assessment complete, you have determined that Clarissa does not have any life-threatening injuries. Her airway, breathing, and circulatory status are stable. Because of the cold conditions, it is best to focus on your patient's injury, splint it, package her, and prepare for transport up the hill.

A patient lying on the frozen ground can become hypothermic, especially if there is any wind. Hypothermia literally means "low temperature." Hypothermia is determined when the core body temperature falls below 95°F (35°C). Below this critical point, the body will no longer be capable of regulating its temperature and the ability to generate heat will diminish. Hypothermia generally goes through four stages. Know how to recognize hypothermia so you can be prepared to treat it before it progresses **Table 8**.

Table 8   Characteristics of Systemic Hypothermia

Core temperature	93° to 95°F (34° to 35°C)	89° to 92°F (32° to 33°C)	80° to 88°F (27° to 31°C)	< 80°F (< 27°C)
Signs and symptoms	Shivering, foot stamping	Loss of coordination, muscle stiffness	Coma	Apparent death
Cardiorespiratory response	Constricted blood vessels, rapid breathing	Slowing respirations, slow pulse	Weak pulse, arrhythmias, very slow respirations	Cardiac arrest
Level of consciousness	Withdrawn	Confused, lethargic, sleepy	Unresponsive	Unresponsive

Keep in mind that it does not need to be below freezing for hypothermia to occur. Signs and symptoms of hypothermia can progress slowly or come on more rapidly, such as when a body is immersed in cold water. When determining if a patient is hypothermic, keep in mind that some patient populations, such as geriatric and pediatric patients, are prone to hypothermia. Patients with the following conditions are also unable to effectively thermoregulate (regulate body heat) and, as a result, are more likely to become hypothermic:

- Trauma, including burns, head injury, or possible injury to the spinal cord
- Shock
- Previously diagnosed medical condition or compromised immune system
- Diabetes
- Hypoglycemia
- Exposure to drugs or toxins

To assess the patient's temperature, pull back on your glove and place the back of your hand or your wrist on the patient's skin at the abdomen. If the skin here feels cool, the patient is likely experiencing hypothermia. Since the weather conditions are less than favorable on this sledding hill, it is imperative that you get your patient packaged and warmed up as soon as possible. Baseline vital signs for a stable patient can wait until your patient is in a warmer environment.

Question 5

What would be the safest way to get your patient to the top of the hill and to the ambulance?

Getting down the hill was just the first step in your patient care. Bringing equipment and an unloaded backboard down a hill is significantly different than carrying the backboard with your patient packaged on it, complete with padded splint, oxygen, and blankets back up the hill.

There is great value in preplanning your lifting and moving. First of all, preplanning will help ensure rescuer safety. Secondly, it will help ensure patient comfort and safety. It is wise, in this situation, to call for lifting and moving assistance from the fire department. Most EMS agencies do not have room on their ambulances to carry or store basket stretchers, while fire departments do. The basket stretcher (sometimes referred to as the Stokes basket or Stokes litter) is designed for use on rough or uneven terrain. Basket stretchers are made either from a durable plastic or a wire or steel frame. The wire basket is very uncomfortable for patients, so padding should be used when placing a patient in this type. Either type of basket is designed to be used to carry patients across fields, over rough terrain, away from cliff edges, and through trails in the woods. Basket stretchers are constructed in a way that allows them to be pulled through water or over snow, with holes in the bottom to allow for drainage. Basket stretchers have also been used in rope rescue situations.

When the fire department is carrying the basket stretcher, as long as they have sufficient personnel, they will usually carry the device with three people per side. This helps to evenly distribute the weight of the patient and makes the load easier on personnel. When moving up the hill, it is best to keep the center of gravity low. Rescuers can do this by traversing the hill or steep incline by going up diagonally instead of straight up. Rescuers run a higher risk of falling if they attempt to go straight up a steep incline.

Patient Care Report for Clarissa

EMS Patient Care Report (PCR)

Date: 03-19-2011	**Incident No.:** 239	**Nature of Call:** Sledding accident	**Location:** North side of Ellison Park
Dispatched: 1502	**En Route:** 1504	**At Scene:** 1515	**Transport:** 1555
At Hospital: 1622	**In Service:** 1648		

Patient Information

Age: 12 years
Sex: Female
Weight (in kg [lb]): 45 kg (100 lb)

Allergies: None
Medications: Children's multivitamin
Past Medical History: None
Chief Complaint: Tibia pain

Vital Signs

Time	BP	Pulse	Respirations	SpO₂
1534	100/68	116 and regular	24 and regular	98% on oxygen
1546	100/66	100 and regular	22 and regular	99% on oxygen

EMS Treatment (circle all that apply)

Oxygen @ 15 L/min via (circle one): NC **(NRM)** Bag-mask device	Assisted Ventilation	Airway Adjunct	CPR
Defibrillation	**Bleeding Control**	**Bandaging**	**(Splinting):** Padded splints to the right lower leg	**(Other):** Spinal immobilization; cold pack to injury site; pain medication

Narrative

Called to Ellison Park (North Hill) for a leg injury due to a sledding accident. Crew was met at the top of the hill by patient's father. Patient was found lying at the base of a tree approximately 30 yards down the hill. Patient's mother and sister were by her side at the time of our arrival. Patient was alert to our presence and complaining of leg pain. Blankets were used immediately for warmth. Airway was patent and breathing appeared unlabored. Chest expansion was equal bilaterally and there was no trauma noted to the chest. Oxygen was applied due to the possibility of internal bleeding. Strong pulses were present in both upper extremities; no visible bleeding; skin was pale, cool, and dry. Initial pain assessment was an 8/10. Focused assessment revealed a swollen, painful, and deformed lower right leg. Pulse, movement, and sensation were positive prior to and after application of padded splints to injured leg. Cold pack wrapped with a cravat placed over injury site prior to splinting. Patient collared, backboarded, and placed in a Stokes basket for transport up the incline, by fire department, to the awaiting and warmed ambulance. ALS medic, Andy, met us on board. Patient's secondary assessment findings were as follows: patient remained alert and oriented for duration of treatment and transport. GCS was 15. Airway was patent and breathing remains unlabored. Respirations were within normal limits with equal chest expansion; no chest trauma was noted and lung sounds were clear; oxygen remained on high flow for duration of transport. Radial pulses remained strong; no bleeding visible anywhere externally; skin was warm, pale, and dry. Abdomen was soft and nontender and there was no pain on palpation. Upper extremities were negative for DCAP-BTLS. Pulse, movement, and sensation were present in all four extremities. Lower left extremity was negative for DCAP-BTLS, with good strong pulse, movement, and sensation. Right lower extremity was swollen, distended, and painful with positive pulse, movement, and sensation. PEARRL. Patient denied hitting her head on impact, and this was confirmed by mom, who witnessed the collision. Patient denied losing consciousness, and this was also confirmed by mom. Patient denied any back, head, or neck pain. En route to Children's Hospital of Wisconsin, patient reported that her pain has decreased to 3/10. Patient triaged to RN Joleeta and moved to trauma bed 1. Side rails up, bed lowered, and patient left in the care of her father and ED staff.
End of report

CASE STUDY 28

Transport Operations

Ambulance Crash at Intersection

You are treating a young woman in the back of the ambulance, heading to Tanner Medical Center. The patient was the victim of an assault on her school campus and sustained a head injury. You are assisting her ventilations and have asked the driver, Peter, to use lights and sirens on the way to the hospital because her condition is deteriorating. You are in the captain's chair (jump seat) and a paramedic, Phil, is on the bench seat. Last night, Peter picked up a shift for a coworker and continued on for his regular shift with you starting at 0700 hours. About 5 minutes out from the hospital, Peter calls in to the emergency department (ED) staff to prepare them for your arrival.

Question 1

What factors can affect the emergency vehicle operator's ability to maintain safe control of the ambulance when traveling with lights and sirens on?

SLAM! Just as Peter finishes his radio transmission, you hear and feel the collision; the ambulance has been struck and is spinning out of control. Peter lets out a loud scream from the front. On impact, your body slams against the cabinets to your right and your head bangs into the hard, plastic door of the top cabinet. A dull thumping sensation unlike anything you have ever felt seems to penetrate your head. The patient slides forward off the gurney and into your left leg near the captain's chair where you were once sitting. The pain you are now feeling in your head and leg is intense.

Question 2

Where do you think most emergency response vehicle crashes take place and why?

When you can finally open your eyes again, you see Phil is still on the bench seat but doubled over in pain. His lap belt is on, but the unsecured cardiac monitor apparently hit him in the abdomen during the impact. With the ambulance on its side, the whole inside of the rig is in utter chaos. The gurney has come loose from the gurney mount, and it, along with your patient, is resting on its side. The patient is lifeless.

For a moment you are too stunned to move. You can hear your heart pounding through your ears. You are relieved to hear Peter on the radio urgently calling for another ambulance to respond to the scene.

Question 3

What could have been done to prevent this crash?

It feels like an eternity passes, even though it has only been a few minutes, when you finally hear sirens coming. Fire trucks, police cars, and ambulances have arrived on scene. You can hear people talking outside as two fire fighters open the back doors. Other medics from your agency appear now that the back doors are safely propped open. Patients are being triaged and, instinctively, you move to help. One of the fire fighters says to you, "Don't get up. We need to get you out of here safely. It looks like you took quite a slam." A colleague is attending to Phil, and another crew is attending to the patient, who is now apneic and pulseless. A few fire fighters and colleagues from your agency have extricated Peter from the cab up front. Four more fire fighters and a paramedic are working on extricating you and Phil from the back of the ambulance.

Once you are immobilized on the backboard, you ask what happened. Apparently, a driver ran the red light and crashed into the side of you at the intersection. "We were so close to the hospital, too," you say. Now that you are out of the wreck, you start to feel the pain searing through your body. Your head is throbbing and the side of your waist feels like someone struck you multiple times with a baseball bat.

Once at the hospital, you are in the trauma bay next to Phil. Peter is three beds down from you. The driver of the car that struck you has been airlifted to Higgins General Hospital. One of the medics who was caring for you tells you that the patient you were transporting has died.

After you undergo computed tomography (CT Scan) to your head and abdomen, the ED physician tells you that you have a small subdural hematoma, a minor laceration to your liver, and a broken right wrist. "It could have been a lot worse, you know," he says. "You weren't wearing your seat belt." "How are Phil and Peter?" you ask anxiously before being taken up to the operating room (OR) for surgery. Peter faired the best due to the location where he was sitting, the use of his seat belt, the deployment of his air bags, and the sound construction of the front cab. Phil was hit pretty hard by the monitor, but his internal bleeding has been contained. He did not lose consciousness and should recover well.

Question 4

What precautions can you take prior to the ambulance moving to ensure safe transport?

Case Analysis

Studies done across several government agencies (including the Centers for Disease Control and Prevention [CDC] and the National Institute for Occupational Safety and Health [NIOSH]) have shown that emergency medical services (EMS) have a high risk of vehicle crashes that include injuries and even fatalities. The risk of occupational death is 2.5 times higher for EMS personnel than for the general working population.[1] From 1991 to 2000 there were 300 fatal crashes involving ambulances that were occupied, which resulted in the deaths of 82 occupants of those ambulances and 275 occupants of other vehicles involved.[2] One study found that during a 10-year period, 72% of occupants killed in crashes involving ambulances were in the back of the ambulance.[3] Many of these EMS providers working in the back of the ambulance during the time of the collision were unrestrained.[4] Some drivers think that if they are driving an emergency response vehicle they are safe. Emergency response drivers may be inexperienced, engage in risky behavior (such as reckless driving), or suffer driver fatigue.

There are many inherent risks to being in the rear compartment of an ambulance. There are few safety standards that exist to protect occupants in the back of ambulances since the patient compartment is largely exempt from the Federal Motor Vehicle Safety Standards (FMVSS). Studies found that the patient compartment is the most dangerous place in the ambulance, in part because fewer than 50% of providers wear seat belts.[5] Often times providers need to remove their seat belts to provide care. For example, cardiopulmonary resuscitation (CPR) in transit is especially dangerous because most people are standing and are not secured in any way. While your hands are occupied during CPR, it is more difficult to brace yourself for sudden stops and moves.

Question 1

What factors can affect the emergency vehicle operator's ability to maintain safe control of the ambulance when traveling with lights and sirens on?

Several factors can affect the emergency vehicle operator's ability to maintain safe control of the ambulance while driving with lights and sirens on, including:
- Driver fatigue: We live in a drowsy society. It is estimated that in the United States alone, people sleep 1.5 hours less than they did just a century ago. One poll in America showed that 63% of adults do not get the recommended 8 hours of sleep every night. Studies have shown that sleep deprivation (both chronic and acute) can have critical effects, both physically and cognitively, on the body. Sleep deprivation can affect alertness, impair memory, impair the immune system, and double the risk of occupational injury. Long-term consequences (chronic) of sleep deprivation include an increase in blood pressure, heart attack, stroke, depression and other mood disorders, and obesity.

---

[1] Thompson, J. March 09, 2009. EMS Providers, CPR Quality "At Risk" During Transport. *EMS1.com*. Available at: http://www.ems1.com/safety/articles/769152-EMS-providers-CPR-quality-at-risk-during-transport/. Accessed July 14, 2011.
[2] Proudfoot, SL. June 2005. Ambulance Crashes: Fatality Factors for EMS Workers. *EMS World*. Available at: http://www.emsworld.com/print/EMS-World/Ambulance-Crashes--Fatality-Factors-for-EMS-Workers/1$1796. Accessed July 14, 2011.
[3] Levick, N. October 2010. Ambulance Safety: Are We Finally Turning a Corner? *EMS World*. Available at: http://www.emsworld.com/print/EMS-World/Ambulance-Safety--/1$14850. Accessed July 14, 2011.
[4] Ibid.
[5] Oriole, K. Fatality Study: EMS Is a Dangerous Profession. *JEMS: Journal of Emergency Medicine*. Available at: http://www.emsedsem.org/Prior%20Articles/EMS_Fatalities%20from%20JEMS.pdf. Accessed July 14, 2011.

The National Highway Traffic Safety Administration (NHTSA) estimates that drowsy driving is responsible for approximately 100,000 automobile crashes, 71,000 injuries, and 1,550 fatalities annually.[6]

- Driver distraction: Any distraction in the cab of the emergency vehicle, which could include music from the radio, radio transmissions, and talking partners, can have an effect on the driver's ability to maintain safe operation of the vehicle.
- Driver drug or alcohol use: Drugs that may impair a driver may be prescription, over-the-counter (OTC), or illegal substances.
- Unqualified emergency response vehicle (ERV) drivers: These drivers can range from those who lack experience (not enough training) to those who have had previous motor vehicle crashes (MVCs) and no remediation after such crashes.
- Other drivers on the road.
- Driving too fast for the conditions.

On the basis of this information, Peter should not have been driving the ambulance after working all night before his shift.

■ Question 2

Where do you think most emergency response vehicle crashes take place and why?

Intersections are where most vehicle collisions occur. In fact, according to the National Highway Traffic Safety Administration (NHTSA), nearly one in five fatal crashes occur at intersections or are intersection related. It is often difficult for other vehicles to see or hear an emergency response vehicle when it is approaching an intersection.

Many of the crashes at intersections involve side impacts to vehicles, where occupants are more vulnerable to critical injury or death. There is very little vehicle protection to the sides of vehicles, compared to that of the front end or rear end. Occupants are less protected during side impacts for several reasons. First, the sides of vehicles (essentially the door panels) are less rigid than the front or rear ends (bumpers). Seat belts provide better protection in front or rear impacts than they do in side impacts. Most vehicles have front air bags; fewer have side air bags. Even when air bags are present, they are designed to work as supplemental safety devices, which work optimally with the use of seat belts. Additionally, a high vehicle (such as an ambulance or SUV) is likely to roll when struck from the side due to its high center of gravity. This leaves occupants more susceptible to serious injury or death.

■ Question 3

What could have been done to prevent this crash?

Although the driver who ran the red light caused the crash, the fatigue of the emergency vehicle driver may have also played a role. It is more difficult to drive defensively if you are fatigued or under the influence of drugs or alcohol. (Chronic fatigue, such as what is found with insomnia or lack of proper sleep, has effects on driving similar to drug or alcohol

---

[6] Breus, MJ. 2004. Chronic Sleep Deprivation May Harm Health. *WebMD*. Available at: http://www.webmd.com/sleep-disorders/guide/important-sleep-habits. Accessed July 14, 2011. Additional information can be found at http://www.sleepdex.org/deficit.htm.

abuse.) Obtaining less than 6 hours of sleep per night affects reaction time, judgment, and coordination.[7]

■ Question 4

What precautions can you take prior to the ambulance moving to ensure safe transport?

In addition to precautions that can be taken while driving, there are many things an EMT can do to ensure safe travel before the ambulance begins moving **Table 1**.

Table 1 Guidelines for Safe Ambulance Driving

1. Select the shortest and least congested route to the scene at the time of the dispatch.
2. Avoid routes with heavy traffic congestion; know alternative routes to each hospital during rush hours.
3. Avoid one-way streets; they may become clogged. Do not go against the flow of traffic on a one-way street, unless absolutely necessary.
4. Watch carefully for bystanders as you approach the scene. Curiosity seekers rarely move out of the way.
5. Park the ambulance in a safe place once you arrive at the scene. If you park facing into traffic, turn off your headlights so that they do not blind oncoming drivers unless they are needed to illuminate the scene. If the vehicle is blocking part of the road, keep your warning lights on to alert oncoming motorists; otherwise, turn them off.
6. Drive within the speed limit while transporting patients, except in the rare extreme emergency.
7. Go with the flow of traffic.
8. Always drive defensively.
9. Always maintain a safe following distance. Use the "4-second rule": Stay at least 4 seconds behind another vehicle in the same lane.
10. Try to maintain an open space or cushion in the lane next to you as an escape route in case the vehicle in front of you stops suddenly.
11. Use your siren if you turn on the emergency lights, except when you are on a freeway.
12. Always assume that other drivers will not hear the siren or see the emergency lights.

Everyone in the ambulance should be securely belted in for safety. This includes patients as well as all EMS providers. Patient restraint use on the gurney should include the use of shoulder straps, not just lap belts. While sitting in the captain's chair, or jump seat, it is easy to be belted in and provide patient care, especially to ventilate a patient because the captain's chair is situated at the cephalic (head) position of the patient. Equipment *must* be secured in all moving ambulances to prevent injury from flying equipment during a crash. Gurney mounts also need to be securely fastened and checked before moving. In the future, ambulance design should take on a more safety-conscious role, such as that now being used in Europe.

---

[7]CNN Staff Writer. September 9, 2000. Sleep Deprivation as Bad as Alcohol Impairment, Study Suggests. *CNN.com*. Available at: http://edition.cnn.com/2000/HEALTH/09/20/sleep.deprivation/. Accessed July 14, 2011.

Patient Care Report for Kazuko

EMS Patient Care Report (PCR)

Date: 04-22-2011	Incident No.: 4563	Nature of Call: Assault	Location: 2115 Campus Drive North		
Dispatched: 0825	En Route: 0827	At Scene: 0838	Transport: 0849	At Hospital:	In Service:

Patient Information

Age: Unobtainable	Allergies: Unobtainable
Sex: Female	Medications: Unobtainable
Weight (in kg [lb]): Unobtainable	Past Medical History: Unobtainable
	Chief Complaint: Unconscious

Vital Signs

Time: 0845	BP: 118/88	Pulse: 100 and irregular	Respirations: 8 and shallow	SpO$_2$: 93% on room air
Time: 0851	BP: 122/90	Pulse: 112 and irregular	Respirations: Assisted at a rate of 10-12 breaths per minute	SpO$_2$: 97% on oxygen
Time:	BP:	Pulse:	Respirations:	SpO$_2$:

EMS Treatment (circle all that apply)

Oxygen @ <u>15</u> L/min via (circle one): NC NRM Bag-mask device	(Assisted Ventilation)	Airway Adjunct	CPR
Defibrillation	Bleeding Control	Bandaging	Splinting	(Other:) Spinal immobilization

Narrative

Responded to a call for a woman who was the victim of an assault on the campus of the community college. Per campus safety, a fellow student heard patient screaming for help and saw a man punching the patient about the head. Assailant ran away when he saw a fellow student running toward them. Campus safety was called as well as 9-1-1. On our arrival, patient was found lying supine on the sidewalk approaching the liberal arts building with campus security present. Patient unresponsive, airway being maintained by Campus Security Officer Caswell. Airway adjunct not used due to gag reflex and the possibility of internal facial trauma. Breathing was inadequate as determined by shallow, slow, and labored breathing at a rate of approximately 8 breaths/min. Chest was negative for DCAP-BTLS. Pulses were irregular; no signs of visible bleeding; skin cool, pale, and moist. Patient collared and immobilized to long board and moved to gurney and then to ambulance. Paramedic Martell met crew at scene and set up equipment in ambulance. Patient's ventilations were assisted throughout duration of treatment and transport. Approximately 5 minutes from Tanner Medical Center, the ambulance, crew, and patient were involved in a motor vehicle collision. The ambulance rolled to its side and the crew was injured. The gurney also came loose from its mount. Responding providers to the scene extricated patient and transported to Tanner Medical Center. **End of report**

CASE STUDY 29

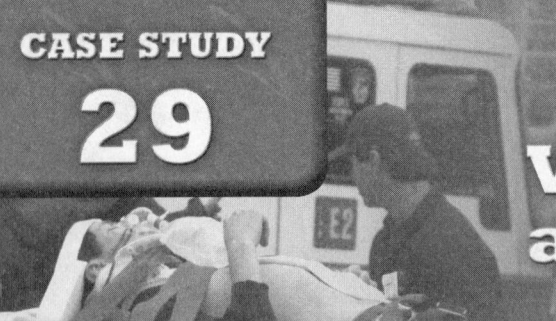

Vehicle Extrication and Special Rescue

Single-Car Motor Vehicle Collision

It is a warm evening in May when you hear the call come in for a single-car motor vehicle collision (MVC). You call your dispatcher to tell him you can take this call with the on-call driver, Scott. As you are heading to the firehouse, you hear an update over the radio: "Police on scene confirm a four-door sedan into a tree on the corner of Whalen Road and County Route 57. It looks like the driver is possibly trapped and not moving. No other vehicles involved."

Question 1

On the basis of the information you currently have for this call, what types of injuries might you suspect in this patient?

Question 2

What clues can you gather from the scene about gaining access and potential injuries before you even make patient contact?

Question 3

How do velocity and mass impact the amount of injury a victim of a motor vehicle collision sustains?

As you and Scott arrive on scene, you get the sense that this crash is going to be challenging. You can see the vehicle crashed into a large oak tree about 25 yards off the main roadway, where you presume the vehicle came from. The oak tree is still standing, but the car has significant front end damage.

Scott parks the ambulance at a safe distance off the shoulder of the road and sets out cones to alert other drivers. Police are on scene and the rescue truck pulls up behind you. Before you approach the vehicle, you look around the scene for clues of how fast the car was moving before hitting the tree. You also look to see if anything fell off the car along the way or if anyone has been ejected. There are some skid marks on the roadway just before the grass, indicating that the driver applied the brakes before the actual collision with the tree. There are also deep ruts in the grass, indicating the car continued on this pathway to the tree.

Nearing the car, you can see the entire front end has been collapsed into the engine compartment. There is significant intrusion damage to this vehicle. You also see that the frame has been bent. You sniff the air to get an idea of whether there is any leaking gasoline coming from the car. You do not see any fluids in the grass on your way to the car.

Approaching the front of the car, or what is left of it, you see the windshield has starring to the driver's side. The driver's side door is also crumpled in. You look in the driver's side window and see there is one occupant, a male who is probably in his early twenties. You walk around to the front passenger side of what is left of the car and yell to the occupant, "Can you hear me, sir?" "Yeah, please help me!" he responds. "My chest and head hurt. It's hard to breathe." You tell him to hold still and you will help him as soon as you can.

Question 4

What type of attire would you wear on a crash scene like this to gain access to and treat this patient?

Question 5

What approach should you take to gain access to this patient?

The rescue truck workers have used cribbing to stabilize the vehicle and disconnected the battery cables. You and Scott go around to the passenger side of the car to try to gain access there. Both doors on this side will not open, despite your attempts at pulling on them. It seems they are jammed due to the crushing of the front end on impact.

Question 6

As the lead EMS provider on this call, what is your primary role right now, since realizing that reaching this patient is going to require complex access? Does this role differ between EMS-based response and fire-based response?

The lieutenant from the rescue truck is now in command of the call. Because you are a trained fire fighter with this fire/rescue agency, you assist in gaining access to this patient. Once the rear passenger side window has been center-punched, and a blanket placed on the frame, Scott climbs in through the window to gain access to your patient. He starts talking to the patient to determine his level of consciousness, covers him with a blanket, and takes head stabilization. Meanwhile, the crew was able to get the front passenger door open and you now also have access to your patient. You do not see anyone else in the vehicle. The young man tells you his name is Justin and he is 23 years old. You perform a quick primary assessment of Justin Table 1.

Vehicle Extrication and Special Rescue

Table 1 — Primary Assessment Findings for Justin

General impression	23-year-old man trapped in car that struck a tree head-on. No seat belt use. Air bags deployed.
Chief complaint	Head and chest pain; difficulty breathing.
Level of consciousness	Alert and oriented to person, place, day, time, and event.
Airway	Patent.
Breathing	Difficulty breathing. Pain on inspiration. Bruising is starting to develop to the chest. Equal expansion bilaterally.
Circulation	Pulses present in carotid and radial. Minor external bleeding to the nose, left cheek, and left forearm.
Life threats	Possible head, neck, spine, and chest injuries.
Pain	Head pain 6 on a scale of 1 to 10. Chest pain 9 on a scale of 1 to 10.
Pertinent negatives	Patient denies loss of consciousness and denies drinking alcohol.
Pupils	Sluggish.
Glasgow coma scale (GCS)	Score: 15 (eye opening, 4; verbal response, 5; motor response, 6).
Interventions	High-flow oxygen applied via nonrebreathing mask (NRM). Cervical spine stabilization. Bleeding controlled with sterile dressings. Rapid extrication.

Question 7

How would you proceed in removing Justin from this vehicle?

Now that the other fire fighters have removed the driver's side door using the hydraulic spreaders, you have the other rescuers bring the backboard over so you can quickly and carefully remove Justin from the vehicle.

With Justin in the back of the rig, you assess baseline vital signs and perform a secondary assessment **Tables 2 and 3**.

Table 2 — Baseline Vital Signs for Justin

Respirations	30 breaths/min and shallow
Pulse rate	119 beats/min and regular
Skin	Cool, pale, and slightly moist
Blood pressure	112/68 mm Hg
Oxygen saturation	96% on oxygen

Table 3	Secondary Assessment Findings for Justin
Level of consciousness	Remains alert and oriented to person, place, day, and event, but now feels "sleepy."
Airway	Remains intact and patent.
Breathing	Difficulty breathing.
	Pain on inspiration.
Circulation	Radial pulse is now weak; carotid pulse still strong and rapid.
	Bleeding has been controlled to the nose, left cheek, and left forearm, as well as to the left knee.
	Skin is pale, moist, and cool.
Head/neck	No pain to the neck.
	Abrasion, bruising, and swelling to the left forehead.
	Patient reporting pain to head.
Chest	Bruising is starting to develop to the left chest wall.
	Flail segment now felt to the left chest wall.
	Bruising noted to the left chest wall with unequal expansion.
	Sternum intact.
	Lung sounds are clear and equal bilaterally.
Abdomen	Some abdominal distention noted to upper quadrants.
	No pain on palpation.
Pelvis/genitalia	Pelvis is intact; no deformities or pain on palpation.
	Patient denies pain to genitalia region, no priapism noted, and no bleeding to genitalia.
Lower extremities	Pulses are weak in the lower extremities.
	Movement and sensation present in both lower extremities.
	Bruising noted to both knees.
Upper extremities	Pulses are weak in the upper extremities.
	Movement and sensation are diminished to the left upper extremity.
	Movement and sensation are positive to the right upper extremity.
Back/neck	Patient denies back and neck pain.
	Difficult to assess DCAP-BTLS to back as patient was rapidly extricated onto the long board.
Pain	Pain to the head remains 6 out of 10.
	Pain to chest remains 9 out of 10.
Glasgow coma scale (GCS)	Score: 14 (eye movement, 4; verbal response, 4; motor response, 6).

You then obtain a SAMPLE history from Justin, including signs and symptoms, allergies, medications, pertinent past medical history, last oral intake, and events leading up to the illness or injury, as you head toward the nearest trauma center Table 4.

Table 4 — SAMPLE History for Justin

Signs and symptoms	Head, neck, and chest trauma due to a single-car MVC into a tree.
	Patient reports chest and head pain.
Allergies	None.
Medications	None.
Pertinent past medical history	Patient denies any medical history.
Last oral intake	Last ate lunch approximately 4 hours ago.
Events leading up to the injury or illness	Driving car on rural road when he lost control and hit a tree head-on.

Based on the mechanism of injury (MOI), you ask Justin some additional history questions (Table 5).

Table 5 — Additional History for Justin

Mechanism of injury	MVC.
Were you wearing your seat belt?	"No."
Do you remember hitting your head on anything?	"Yes, I think I hit it on the windshield and maybe the side window."
Do you know how fast you were going at the time of the crash?	"Uh, I don't know. Maybe 55 mph."
Did you lose consciousness today?	"No."

Advanced life support (ALS) meets with you en route to the trauma center for fluid replacement and further evaluation. As you assess another set of vital signs (Table 6), Scott calls ahead to let the trauma center know you are coming in.

Table 6 — Second Set of Vital Signs for Justin

Respirations	10–12 breaths/min assisted via bag-valve mask (BVM)
Pulse rate	114 beats/min and regular
Skin	Cool, pale, and slightly moist
Blood pressure	100/62 mm Hg
Oxygen saturation	97% with assisted ventilations and high-flow oxygen

Question 8

What pertinent scene information do you need to share with the emergency department staff at the hospital? Why?

Case Analysis

Question 1

On the basis of the information you currently have for this call, what types of injuries might you suspect in this patient?

The extent of injury will depend, in part, on whether the driver or occupants used seat belts, if the vehicle has air bags, and if the air bags deployed. With that said, the MOIs and the condition of the interior of the vehicle give you clues as to what injuries you are likely to find in your patient.

In MVCs there are usually three types of impact. There is the impact of the vehicle into an object—for example, a tree or utility pole. Then, there is a collision of the occupants inside the vehicle against the interior of the passenger compartment. The third collision occurs inside the patient's body when the internal organs strike against solid structures of the body, such as bones and other organs. In the thoracic cage, for example, the heart may strike against the sternum, with the resulting injury being a torn or ruptured aorta, which may cause fatal bleeding. Other types of injuries may include:

- Knees can strike the dashboard causing lower extremity (femur fracture, for example) and pelvic injuries.
- Potentially serious chest and abdominal injuries can occur from striking the steering wheel.
- Facial abrasions and even epistaxis (nosebleed) can result from air bag deployment.
- Head and spinal injuries can result when the face and head strike the windshield.
- Passengers in the back can also be seriously injured, especially if they are not properly secured with a seat belt. Their heads can strike the side windows, and intrusion from a lateral impact can cause injury to the side of the body.
- If passengers are not restrained, regardless of their seating position, they may be partially ejected or ejected from the vehicle.
- Rear-end impacts tend to cause whiplash-type injuries, especially when the head and/or neck is not restrained by a headrest.
- Lateral collisions (oftentimes referred to as t-bone collisions) typically strike the vehicle above its center of gravity from a side impact. This tends to cause a type of whiplash that pulls the passenger's shoulders and head toward the intruding vehicle or object, causing much lateral movement to the spine.
- Rollover crashes are most harmful to those passengers who are not restrained. The passenger who is unrestrained can have multiple strikes within the vehicle during the rollover process. The most dangerous element of rollover crashes is ejection from a motor vehicle. The ejected passenger may hit any of a number of items before, during, and after ejection.

Question 2

What clues can you gather from the scene about gaining access and potential injuries before you even make patient contact?

The type of damage to the vehicle gives crucial information about the MOI and possibly the severity of injury to the occupants. Depending on the type of impact, there are many questions you can ask yourself when approaching the scene of an MVC, such as:

- Are the tires deflated?
- Are the windows intact, in particular the windshield?
- Are there tree limbs down around the vehicle?
- Are there any electrical wires down near the vehicle or in the path that the vehicle took?
- Does it look like the car overturned?
- Do I see or smell smoke?
- Is the frame bent?
- In what position is the vehicle situated?
- Are there any obstructions in the way of accessing the patient in the vehicle?
- Is there air-bag deployment?
- Is there passenger compartment intrusion?
- Are any other vehicles involved?
- Did any part of a tree fall on the car, causing additional impact?
- How many patients might there be?
- Are there skid marks showing that the vehicle attempted to brake prior to impact?
- Is this a high-speed area?
- What size vehicle is it?
- What are the road conditions?
- Does the severity of damage prevent my access to patients?
- What are the weather conditions?
- Do I see any fluids leaking from the vehicle?

Question 3

How do velocity and mass impact the amount of injury a victim of a motor vehicle collision sustains?

As you know, the MOI is how the patient got hurt. Kinetic energy reflects the relationship between the mass (weight) of the object and the velocity (speed) at which it is traveling. Kinetic energy is calculated as follows:

$$\text{Kinetic energy} = \frac{\text{Mass} \times \text{Velocity}^2}{2}$$

Mass equals the weight of an object, while velocity equals the speed of an object. The heavier the moving object, the higher the velocity, or speed, of that object. The faster a vehicle travels and then crashes, the higher the amount of energy that was absorbed in that vehicle, including any persons in that vehicle. Thus the kinetic energy can indicate the severity of the MOI.

Question 4

What type of attire would you wear on a crash scene like this to gain access to and treat this patient?

To gain access to a motor vehicle that has crashed and sustained significant damage, it is important to wear proper attire to avoid injury. Suitable attire would include a turnout coat, leather work gloves, a helmet, boots, and bunker pants. A standard-issue EMS uniform is not appropriate for entering a car involved in a crash due to the possibility of encountering broken glass, plastic, or metal.

Question 5

What approach should you take to gain access to this patient?

Simple access is a good place to start when attempting to gain access to a patient. In this case, trying all the doors would be a good place to start because it does not require any special tools. EMTs working with an EMS-only agency should not approach the vehicle until it has been stabilized by the fire department. Park at a safe distance from the crash scene. Choose a location that will allow for effective traffic control and will maximize scene safety for your crew, responding agencies, and the patient. Generally speaking, it is good practice to park about 100′ past the scene on the same side of the road. It is also advisable to park uphill and upwind from the scene in case any smoke or hazardous materials are involved in the crash scene. Leave your ambulance's warning lights turned on when you park at the crash scene. Parking in this manner will provide you and other responders with a cushion of space between your emergency vehicle and operations at the scene. Be alert to any hazards that might cause a fire, explosive hazards, downed wires, and any structures that might collapse into the scene or onto your emergency vehicle.

Question 6

As the lead EMS provider on this call, what is your primary role right now, since realizing that reaching this patient is going to require complex access? Does this role differ between EMS-based response and fire-based response?

If you are with an EMS-based unit and have no fire or rescue training, your role as lead EMS provider is to stand by, in a safe location near the car, and wait for the fire department to gain access to the patient. During this time, you may ask for updates on your patient and be prepared with the necessary equipment. If you are with a fire or rescue department, you may be asked to assist in the rescue operation until access has been obtained.

Question 7

How would you proceed in removing Justin from this vehicle?

There are generally two options for removing patients from vehicles when you are concerned about trauma to the spine. The first is to use a vest-type immobilization device (or similar). Using this type of immobilization device takes a little bit of time and may not be suitable for patients who require immediate removal from the vehicle due to complications (such as a compromised airway or uncontrolled bleeding). The other option is to rapidly extricate the patient onto a backboard. This will involve a minimum of three people to move this patient from the seat of the car to the backboard while maintaining in-line spinal stabilization.

Question 8

What pertinent scene information do you need to share with the emergency department staff at the hospital? Why?

Considering the fact that the emergency department staff was not on scene, you need to give them a good sense of what the scene was like so they have an idea of the severity or potential severity of the patient's condition.

For example, if a patient fell down a full flight of concrete steps to the concrete cellar floor, the potential for injury would be much greater than if the patient fell down two steps and injured an ankle. Telling the triage nurse that the patient merely "fell" on the steps does not give a full and accurate picture of what really happened. The same holds true for an MVC. If a vehicle was rear-ended at a low speed (less than 25 mph) in a parking lot, this is significantly different than a car that was rear-ended at a stoplight by another car traveling at a high rate of speed (greater than 40 mph).

It will be helpful for the hospital staff to know:
- Was the patient wearing a seat belt?
- Were air bags deployed?
- How much intrusion damage was there, if any?
- Were any other occupants involved? If so, what is their condition?
- Was the windshield intact?
- Was there damage to the steering column?
- Was there any external blood loss? Is so, estimate by looking at the upholstery of the vehicle or the surroundings?
- Were there any skid marks?
- How much damage was there to the vehicle?
- Were there any other vehicles involved? If so, what type of vehicles were they? Sub-compact car, compact car, full-sized sedan, mini-van, utility truck, tractor trailer, motorcycle, bus?

This descriptive information will give the hospital staff a clear picture of what happened to your patient and a better idea of the potential extent of injuries.

Patient Care Report for Justin

EMS Patient Care Report (PCR)

Date: 05-12-2010	Incident No.: 546	Nature of Call: MVC		Location: Whalen Road and Rte. 57	
Dispatched: 1912	En Route: 1914	At Scene: 1925	Transport: 1952	At Hospital: 2009	In Service: 2040

Patient Information

Age: 23 years
Sex: Male
Weight (in kg [lb]): 96 kg (212 lb)

Allergies: None
Medications: None
Past Medical History: None
Chief Complaint: Chest and head pain, difficulty breathing

Vital Signs

Time	BP	Pulse	Respirations	SpO$_2$
1940	112/68	119 and regular	30 and shallow	96% on oxygen
1947	100/62	114 and regular	Assisting ventilations	97% with assisted ventilations and oxygen

EMS Treatment (circle all that apply)

Oxygen @ **15** L/min via (circle one): NC (NRM) (Bag-mask device)	(Assisted Ventilation) 10-12 per minute	Airway Adjunct	CPR
Defibrillation	(Bleeding Control) 4 × 4's used to control bleeding to face and forearm	(Bandaging) Bulky dressing to flail segment	Splinting	(Other:) spinal immobilization

Narrative

Responded to call for single-car MVC with a four-door sedan into a tree off the roadway in a 55 mph zone. No other vehicles involved. Significant front end damage to the vehicle was noted (front end crumpled into the engine compartment). Patient was driver of vehicle and reported he was not wearing his seat belt and air bags did deploy. Rescue company stabilized vehicle and gained access to the patient via the driver's side door using hydraulic spreaders. EMT Scott entered the vehicle to hold head stabilization while the patient was being accessed. Patient initially presented as follows: alert and oriented with a patent airway; difficulty breathing, pain on inspiration, bruising to anterior chest wall with equal chest expansion; carotid and radial pulses present and strong, skin was pale, cool, and moist; minor bleeding to the nose, left cheek, and left forearm. Oxygen initially given via NRM at 15 L/min while patient still in car. Patient stated he was going "about 55 mph" when he went off the road. Patient denied loss of consciousness and denied drinking alcohol. Patient stated he last ate at lunchtime. Pulse, movement, and sensation were positive when assessed prior to application of cervical collar. Bleeding controlled to the face and forearm, and patient rapidly extricated from vehicle as his level of consciousness was declining and his pain and difficulty breathing were increasing. Paramedic unit 52 on scene and on board for transport. Secondary assessment revealed the following: patient presented with altered level of consciousness and reported feeling "sleepy" with increased difficulty in following commands. Airway remained intact, no oropharyngeal airway used due to gag reflex, and no nasopharyngeal airway used due to facial trauma and potential head trauma. Breathing remained labored with pain on inspiration. Chest rise was asymmetrical with good chest rise on the right and diminished chest rise on the left, and flail segment now felt on left side with increased bruising. Flail segment stabilized with bulky dressings and taped in place. Radial pulses weak; carotid pulse strong and rapid. No jugular vein distension noted, no tracheal deviation, and no c-spine deformities noted prior to placing the collar. Patient reported pain to head rated as 6/10; abrasion, bruising, and swelling noted to the left forehead; pupils were sluggish to respond but respond equally. Lung sounds were clear and equal bilaterally. Pain to chest rated as 9/10. Sternum was intact, and paradoxical movement to the chest wall was noted. Some abdominal distention was noted to the upper quadrants; no pain on palpation and no rigidity. No distention to the lower quadrants and no rigidity. Pelvis was intact. Patient denied pain to genitalia, and no priapism noted. Pulses were weak in the lower extremities, movement and sensation were present in both lower extremities, and bruising was noted to both knees. Pulses were weak in the upper extremities, and movement and sensation were diminished to the left upper extremity. Movement and sensation were positive in the right upper extremity. Patient denied back and neck pain. Difficult to assess back due to rapid extrication. Assisted patient's ventilations at a rate of 10-12 breaths per minute en route to Mercy Medical Center. Crew greeted by trauma team and immediately escorted to trauma bay 1. Moved patient on backboard over to bed with bed railings placed up. Gave report to Dr. Ververs and Dr. Michaels. **End of report**

CASE STUDY 30

Incident Management

Fire Fighter Rehab at Working Fire

You and your partner, Marshall, are driving through the city waiting for the next emergency medical services (EMS) call to come in. The EMS channel is oddly quiet for the moment. You hope it stays that way, as the temperature is hovering around 90°F (32.2°C) with the humidity around 90%. Just then, you hear the fire dispatcher come across the radio with a working fire in an apartment complex: "Dispatch to Battalion 3 for a working residential fire at 160 Bay Street, between Avenue C and Castle Street, box 353. Engine 10, Engine 16, Rescue 11, Quint Midi 6, and Battalion Chief to respond." You decide to head toward the vicinity, which is about eight blocks to the east. As you are heading over, dispatch updates you that the first engine on scene confirms a working fire, with possible trapped residents.

Question 1
Where can you find guidelines for emergency incident rehab?

Question 2
What is the rationale for fire fighter rehab?

Question 3
What are your responsibilities during emergency incident rehabilitation?

Question 4
Describe the functions of the rehabilitation sectors.

You arrive on scene and find the incident commander (IC). He tells you to head around the corner to help set up the rehab sector. As Marshall drives around the corner, you see that the fire safety officer, Captain Fitch, has already begun setting up a rehab sector in a portable tent. Captain Fitch asks you to assist in setting up folding chairs, blankets, fans, water bottles, and other essential monitoring equipment. A portable generator off the rescue truck has also been set up.

Question 5

As EMS personnel on the scene, what medical monitoring and assessing should you be responsible for?

Question 6

Describe some of the inherent threats to the health and safety of fire fighters at a working fire.

Question 7

Who is responsible for sending fire fighters to rehab?

About 45 minutes after your arrival on scene, three fire fighters enter the rehab sector, log in, and remove their gear. Your patient is a fire fighter named Dale. You assess Dale's baseline vital signs **Table 1**.

Table 1 Baseline Vital Signs for Dale

Respirations	26 breaths/min and regular
Pulse	122 beats/min, strong and regular
Skin	Flushed, warm, and moist
Blood pressure	156/90 mm Hg
Oxygen saturation	97%
Temperature	100.4°F/38°C tympanic

Given the heat, humidity, and stress level of this working fire, you are not surprised by these vital signs. There are two fans set up at your station and three additional large fans at the medical evaluation/treatment area. You have also set up forearm immersion tubs to accelerate core temperature cooling.

Question 8

What medical conditions should you be concerned about when assessing fire fighters in rehab?

Now that baseline vitals have been established, you encourage Dale to replenish his fluids, which he does eagerly, while you conduct a primary assessment **Table 2**.

Incident Management

Table 2 — Primary Assessment Findings for Dale

General impression	38-year-old male fire fighter in rehab at working structure fire.
Chief complaint	None.
Level of consciousness	Alert and oriented to person, place, time, and event.
Airway	Patent.
Breathing	Breathing is shallow.
	Chest expansion is equal bilaterally.
	Lung sounds clear.
Circulation	Radial pulse is strong, rapid, and regular.
	Skin is warm, flushed, and moist.
Life threats	Possibility of heat exhaustion.
Pain	None.
Pertinent negatives	Patient denies difficulty breathing and chest pain.
	No trauma to the chest.
	No external bleeding noted anywhere.
	Patient denies loss of consciousness.
Pupils	Pupils are equal, round, regular in size, and react properly to light (PEARRL).
Glasgow coma scale (GCS)	Score: 15 (eye opening, 4; verbal response, 5; motor response, 6).
Interventions	Monitor vital signs.
	Passive cooling with removal of protective gear (helmet, bunker coat, etc).

Question 9

What should you monitor in the fire fighter while he is resting, cooling down, and replenishing his fluids?

It has been about 10 minutes since you assessed baseline vital signs, so you obtain a second set of vital signs for Dale **Table 3**.

Table 3 — Second Set of Vital Signs for Dale

Respirations	22 breaths/min and regular
Pulse	110 beats/min, strong and regular
Skin	Flushed, warm, and dry
Blood pressure	152/88 mm Hg
Oxygen saturation	97%
Temperature	99.5°F/37.5°C tympanic

The vital signs for two of the fire fighters in rehab, Rich and Scott, have come down to acceptable levels and their medical assessment is within normal limits, so they are released from rehab. Dale's vital signs, however, have not come down yet. Following the NFPA 1584 standards for fire fighter rehab, Dale stays in rehab for another 20 minutes of rest, further oral hydration, and implementation of active cooling methods using cool, wet towels placed on his neck. While Dale is cooling off, you obtain a SAMPLE history from him, including signs and symptoms, allergies, medications, pertinent past medical history, last oral intake, and events leading up to the injury or illness **Table 4**.

Table 4 SAMPLE History for Dale

Signs and symptoms	Headache and feeling light-headed after being in rehab for over 40 minutes.
Allergies	Penicillin.
Medications	Loratadine as needed for seasonal allergies.
Pertinent past medical history	No medical history other than the seasonal allergies.
Last oral intake	Fluid and carbohydrate replacement at rehab approximately 15 minutes ago.
Events leading up to the injury or illness	Fighting structure fire as interior fire fighter for approximately 30 minutes.
	Ordered to rehab after a 30-minute self-contained breathing apparatus (SCBA) cylinder was emptied.

Dale tells you that he feels light-headed and reports a headache, which is cause for further evaluation on your part. Upon questioning, Dale tells you that he is nauseated and is starting to have mild chest pressure. These are parameters for transporting to a hospital for further medical evaluation. After having him lie down and providing high-flow oxygen, you confer with the Incident Commander (IC), who agrees that Dale needs to be transported to Wilmington General. You call for a paramedic to accompany you and your patient to the hospital. En route, you perform a secondary assessment **Table 5**.

Incident Management

Table 5 Secondary Assessment Findings for Dale

Level of consciousness	Remains alert and oriented to person, place, day, time, and event, but feels light-headed.
Airway	Open and patent.
Breathing	Unlabored, but shallow. Chest expansion remains equal bilaterally. Lung sounds are clear.
Circulation	Skin is flushed, warm, and dry. Pulses are strong and rapid.
Head/neck	No DCAP-BTLS noted. No jugular vein distension (JVD) or trachea deviation.
Chest	No chest trauma. No scars noted.
Abdomen	Soft, nontender, no pain on palpation.
Pelvis/genitalia	Pelvis is intact and without pain. No pain or swelling in genitalia.
Lower extremities	Lower extremities are negative for DCAP-BTLS. Pulse, movement, and sensation are positive in both lower extremities.
Upper extremities	Upper extremities are negative for DCAP-BTLS. Pulse, movement, and sensation are positive in both upper extremities.
Back/neck	No DCAP-BTLS noted in back or neck. No pain to back or neck.
Life threats	Hyperthermia.
Pain	Headache 6 on a scale of 1 to 10.
Pertinent negatives	No external bleeding anywhere.
Pupils	PEARRL
Glasgow coma scale (GCS)	Score: 15 (eye opening, 4; verbal response, 5; motor response, 6).
Interventions	Oxygen on high flow (15 L/pm) via nonrebreathing mask (NRM). Cold packs are placed at the armpits, groin area, and back of neck for active cooling.

Once at Wilmington General, you give patient information to registered nurse (RN) Harry and move Dale to trauma bed 2. Bed rails are up and the bed is lowered. Dr. Chandaroy gets pertinent patient information from you before you leave. You wish Dale a speedy recovery and wash your hands before heading out to clean up the ambulance and start your documentation.

Question 10

Explain documentation procedures for the emergency incident rehabilitation report.

Case Analysis

■ Question 1

Where can you find guidelines for emergency incident rehab?

The National Fire Protection Association (NFPA) was established in 1896 and is an international, nonprofit organization. According to the organization, they are the world's leading advocate for fire prevention and an authoritative resource on public safety. NFPA 1584, "Standard on the Rehabilitation Process for Members During Emergency Operations and Training Exercises," is a policy and guideline for fire fighter and responder rehabilitation. Check on local protocols regarding fire fighter and responder rehab operating procedures in your state or region.

■ Question 2

What is the rationale for fire fighter rehab?

Fire fighter and responder rehab is needed to help prevent any injury or illness to fire fighters and emergency responders on the scene of, for example, a working fire. Strenuous physical exertion, like fighting a fire, has been found to cause significant cardiac episodes. The most common cause of fire fighter death is not from fires, but from cardiac arrest secondary to heat and exertion. Recent statistics show that cardiac events were responsible for 45% of fire fighter line-of-duty deaths. Rehabilitation in the fire and EMS sector is designed to diminish the effects of stress during firefighting (or working at mass-casualty incidents or other hazardous scenes). Another goal is to help enable the member to return to work while decreasing the chances of on-scene injury, diminished health, or death. Rehabilitation, as set forth by the NFPA 1584 guidelines, is an organized intervention to care for working members of the organization (fire fighters and/or EMS personnel).

■ Question 3

What are your responsibilities during emergency incident rehabilitation?

Generally speaking, if you are an EMS agency being called in to perform rehab functions, you will be responsible for medical monitoring. This may include monitoring vital signs and providing refreshments, medical evaluation, and transport. Part of your responsibilities may include ensuring appropriate equipment is available for medical monitoring. This may include, but is not limited to:

- Thermometers
- Oxygen
- Oxygen delivery equipment (masks, tubing, etc)
- Airway supplies
- Blankets
- Pulse oximeter
- Carbon monoxide monitor
- Automated external defibrillator (AED)
- Bleeding control supplies
- Orthopaedic injury supplies (splints, etc)
- Seating
- Stretchers

- Towels
- Handwashing supplies
- Cardiac medications (such as aspirin/ASA)
- ECG monitor (for ALS providers)
- Other medical supplies, such as blood pressure cuffs, stethoscopes, pen lights

■ Question 4

Describe the functions of the rehabilitation sectors.

The functions of the rehab sectors are as follows:
- **Accountability/log-in/log-out:** This ensures proper documentation and tracking of personnel entering and exiting the rehab area.
- **Gear/storage area:** This is primarily a location for self-contained breathing apparatus (SCBA) exchange (old cylinders are traded in for new ones).
- **Vital sign monitoring/determination:** Vital signs are assessed in this area and recorded for trending purposes as well as for clearance back into the field.
- **Rest/refreshment area:** Fire fighters should rehydrate and replenish here. Noncaffeinated, noncarbonated, low-sugar, nonfructose beverages, such as water and electrolyte liquids, are provided. Foods should include carbohydrates (fruits, vegetables, and grains), proteins, and fats in smaller, more frequent meals.
- **Medical evaluation/treatment area:** This area is for monitoring members who are at risk of suffering adverse health or safety ramifications. Vital sign monitoring will be done here as well. It is in this area that a determination will be made regarding the following:
  - The need for immediate transport to the hospital
  - Close monitoring and treatment
  - Release from rehab back into the field
- **Transportation assignment:** A transportation unit leader will determine where the fire fighter will be transported to and by which ambulance.

■ Question 5

As EMS personnel on scene, what medical monitoring and assessing should you be responsible for?

Most often, EMS personnel on the scene of a rehab unit will monitor vital signs and evaluate the overall physical well-being of the fire fighter. If a fire fighter needs further treatment, you may also be called upon to transport him or her to the hospital.

■ Question 6

Describe some of the inherent threats to the health and safety of fire fighters at a working fire.

With the use of SCBA, the frequency of smoke inhalation has decreased over the years. However, other hazards still exist, such as heat exhaustion. Firefighting can be an extremely physical job and can put stress on the body. Personal protective equipment (PPE), along with the extreme temperatures of fire, can lead to overexertion and overheating of fire fighters. Falls are a risk as well, especially from ladders, rooftops, and unstable surfaces. Working on the side of roadways is also an inherent hazard of working as a fire fighter or EMT. Drivers are often distracted and do not always see the EMS and fire personnel working in or near roadways.

■ Question 7

Who is responsible for sending fire fighters to rehab?

This may vary slightly by each organization's standard operating procedure (SOP) or standard operating guideline (SOG). Generally speaking, it is the responsibility of the IC or company officers to send fire fighters to rehab. EMS personnel provide feedback and suggestions but usually do not have the authority to keep a fire fighter in rehab. This is where good communication comes into play. If you recognize there is a potential problem, like vital signs not coming back to normal or a change in level of consciousness, then communicate with the rehab manager.

■ Question 8

What medical conditions should you be concerned about when assessing fire fighters in rehab?

Heat exhaustion (marked by increased body temperature), changes in level of consciousness, cold stress, heart attack, respiratory distress, and/or hypertension despite rehab efforts are just some of the medical conditions you should be on the lookout for during fire fighter rehab.

■ Question 9

What should you monitor in the fire fighters while he is resting, cooling down, and replenishing his fluids?

Vital signs including temperature, pulse, respirations, and blood pressure should be assessed. In addition, watch for changes in level of consciousness.

■ Question 10

Explain documentation procedures for the emergency incident rehabilitation report.

Medical monitoring needs to be documented; however, this documentation will be kept separately from medical treatment records. Rehab tags or charts can help keep track of personnel trends and initial documentation **Figure 1**. Vital sign trending, level of alertness, any signs associated with cold or heat stress, fluid replacement, and whether active cooling took place are all examples of medical monitoring items to document. If personnel are then transported for further evaluation, a standard PCR should be completed when transported.

SAMPLE REHAB TAG

Date: _____ Name: _____

Log-in Time: ____:____ Log-out Time: ____:____

Age: _____ Sex: _____M _____F Company: _____

Weather Conditions

Temperature	Wind Chill	Wet	Index

Vital Signs on Entry

Time	BP	Pulse	Respirations	Temperature
To Enter Medical	Systolic < 90 or > 160 Diastolic > 110	> 120		> 99.5°F

☐ REHAB ONLY
☐ MEDICAL EVAL AND REHAB

Vital Signs Assessed Every 10 Minutes

			Retain for Further Rehab/Tx
Time			
BP			> 160 S < 100 S > 90 D
Pulse			> 100
Resp.			
Temp.			> 99.5°F
Assessed by:			

Symptoms/Comments

Disposition

☐ Return to fire ground/scene   ☐ Off duty   ☐ Transport to hospital

Rehab Officer:

Time Released:

Figure 1 Sample Rehab Tag.

Patient Care Report for Dale

EMS Patient Care Report (PCR)

Date: 08-12-2010	Incident No.: 104536	Nature of Call: Fire Standby		Location: 160 Bay Street	
Dispatched: 1725	En Route: 1725	At Scene: 1729	Transport: 1850	At Hospital: 1912	In Service: 1935

Patient Information

Age: 38 years	Allergies: Penicillin
Sex: Male	Medications: Loratadine as needed for seasonal allergies
Weight (in kg [lb]): 74 kg (165 lb)	Past Medical History: Seasonal allergies
	Chief Complaint: Light-headed, headache

Vital Signs

Time	BP	Pulse	Respirations	SpO$_2$
1815	156/90	122, strong and regular	26 and shallow	97% on room air
1826	152/88	110, strong and regular	22 and regular	97% on room air

EMS Treatment (circle all that apply)

Oxygen @ **15** L/min via (circle one): NC **(NRM)** Bag-mask device	Assisted Ventilation	Airway Adjunct	CPR
Defibrillation	Bleeding Control	Bandaging	Splinting	**(Other:)** Active cooling using cool, wet towels to the neck

Narrative

Crew called to assist with fire fighter rehab at working structure fire. Patient was ordered to rehab after his 30-minute SCBA tank was depleted. Initial assessment revealed the following: patient was alert and oriented with a patent airway. Breathing was shallow, lung sounds were clear, and there was equal expansion of the chest bilaterally; there was no trauma to the chest; radial pulses were strong, rapid, and regular; skin was warm, flushed, and moist; there was no external bleeding anywhere. Initial tympanic temperature was 100.4°F/38°C. At time of initial assessment, patient had no chief complaints. Patient was in rehab for approximately 30 minutes, and both passive and active cooling techniques were used to bring core body temperature down (removal of turnout coat, helmet, gloves; cooling with fans; moist towels to the neck). After assessing second set of vital signs and oral fluid and carbohydrate intake, patient's temperature remained high and vital signs remained out of the normal range. Second tympanic temperature was 99.5°F/37.5°C. Patient also began to complain of feeling light-headed and having a headache. Head pain was a 6/10. Patient was assisted into a supine position on a rehab cot, ALS was contacted, and rehab commander was notified of changes to patient. Crew advised patient and rehab commander that patient should be transported. Patient moved to stretcher and then to awaiting rig for ALS transport to Wilmington General Hospital. Bunker pants and shirt were removed and a secondary assessment was performed, which revealed the following: patient was still conscious and alert but feeling light-headed; head pain remained a 6/10. Airway was patent; breathing was unlabored but shallow, with patient on high-flow oxygen via NRM; chest expansion remained equal bilaterally and lung sounds were clear; no trauma to the chest and no scars noted. Skin was still flushed, warm, and dry; pulses were strong and rapid. There was no external bleeding anywhere. Head and neck were without DCAP-BTLS; no JVD or trachea deviation. Abdomen was soft, nontender; pelvis was intact and without pain; genitalia were without pain or swelling. Upper and lower extremities were without DCAP-BTLS, and all four extremities were positive for pulse, movement, and sensation. There was no pain or DCAP-BTLS to the back or neck. GCS was a 15. Cold packs were placed at the armpits, groin area, and back of neck for active cooling. ALS transport to hospital was otherwise unremarkable. Patient triaged to RN Harry and moved to bed 2 in the trauma bay. Bed rails left up, bed lowered to lowest position, and patient left in the care of the ED staff. **End of report**

CASE STUDY 31

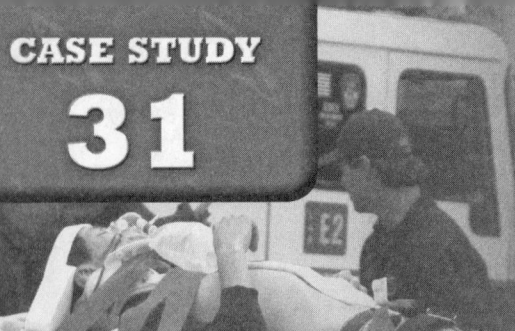

Terrorism Response and Disaster Management

Illnesses of Unknown Cause Reported at the Airport

It is the day before Thanksgiving when you and your driver, Stephanie, receive a call to the airport for a couple who are feeling ill. They are in the west terminal, Concourse A, near security. Given the upcoming holiday, you know the airport will be crowded. En route, you hear the emergency medical services (EMS) dispatcher over the air. This call is also for a person who is ill at the airport—a 21-year-old man in the west terminal, Concourse D. Another unit from within the district responds to the call. Just as you approach the ramp to enter the terminal, the dispatcher is on the air with a third call for a family who is ill at the airport. The family is also located in the west terminal, Concourse A.

Question 1

Are these simultaneously occurring illnesses a coincidence?

Question 2

Given your suspicions, how do you think you should approach this scene? Should you proceed to the area to which you were called? Why or why not?

Question 3

What resources might you call to assist with this situation?

After hearing subsequent calls for the illnesses at the airport in the same terminal, you and Stephanie shoot each other a concerned look. You decide not to stop near the entrance and instead head for safety on a perimeter road just east of the entrance. As Stephanie drives off the airport property, you call the dispatcher with your concerns about these calls. The other unit will also divert until further notice. The dispatcher sends an update that they have now received several calls for the same type of illness in the west terminal, Concourse A.

The dispatcher instructs you and other responding agencies to turn all radio transmissions to frequency 175.5, a dedicated frequency for this incident. You receive the following updates from the dispatcher:

1. People in the main lobby of the airport have not reported any signs or symptoms of illness yet.
2. Five security guards in the west terminal, Concourse A, are now reporting similar illnesses.
3. Some of the signs and symptoms reported by victims include runny nose, watery eyes and eye pain, drooling and excessive sweating, cough, rapid breathing, nausea, vomiting, headache, drowsiness, and confusion.
4. The airport fire department has set up a command post on the east side of the airport, which is currently upwind of the main airport and west terminal.
5. Local law enforcement is working with the Transportation Security Administration (TSA). TSA has secured the east end terminal as well as the front lobby. They are not allowing anyone to enter or exit these areas. All departing flights have been grounded, and incoming flights are being diverted to the nearest airport. As unsuspecting travelers are entering the airport property, local law enforcement is diverting them. Aside from necessary responders, no one is allowed on or off the airport property.
6. Air traffic control is in contact with the pilots on the grounded airplanes, inquiring as to whether anyone on board the planes is either feeling ill or behaving suspiciously.
7. All of the responding EMS agencies are now at a staging area awaiting further instructions.

As you listen to the radio and await further instructions, you take out the US Department of Transportation's *Emergency Response Guidebook* to see if you can pinpoint what type of agent may be causing the signs and symptoms of the victims inside the airport Figure 1.

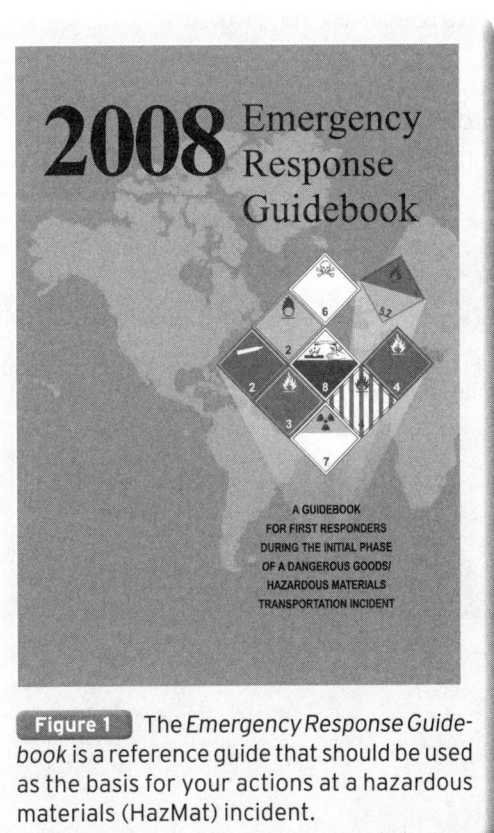

Figure 1 The *Emergency Response Guidebook* is a reference guide that should be used as the basis for your actions at a hazardous materials (HazMat) incident.

Question 4

On the basis of the signs and symptoms you were provided, what are the possibilities for the type of agent used?

A hazardous materials (HazMat) team has entered the building and is giving more updates. They believe the substance may have come from the air ducts in the terminal. They are investigating the source to try to analyze what agent it may be. Reports are now coming in that the HazMat team is setting up decontamination areas outside on the ground near the affected terminals. EMS is being asked to line up ambulances outside the decontamination area to receive victims. The EMS Operations Commander has made the local hospitals aware of the situation and informed them that EMS providers may be transporting patients to local facilities soon.

Question 5

What are weapons of mass destruction (WMDs)?

Question 6

Why are the mnemonics SLUDGEM and DUMBELS used? What does each letter stand for?

Question 7

What is the EMT's role in a potential terrorism event?

Follow-up with the HazMat team reveals that the agent tabun (GA), a chemical warfare nerve agent, was discovered in the airport's west terminal. As you and Stephanie wait in the decontamination area to receive your first patient, you are grateful that you did not enter the building for this call.

Question 8

What are some special considerations when dealing with mass-casualty incidents (MCIs), particularly those that involve a decontamination zone?

Case Analysis

■ Question 1

Are these simultaneously occurring illnesses a coincidence?

When numerous people report similar illnesses or signs and symptoms of illness, this should be cause for concern. For example, a family in a single household may report that they are feeling ill. Could it be a virus or bacterial infection, or could it be carbon monoxide poisoning? Until proven otherwise, use your gut instinct and caution when approaching these situations. In this particular scenario, it does seem odd that so many people located at the airport would fall ill at the same time within a concentrated area. For safety purposes, always be cautious and alert before entering the scene.

■ Question 2

Given your suspicions, how do you think you should approach this scene? Should you proceed to the area to which you were called? Why or why not?

If you have been made aware of other calls reporting similar signs and symptoms from people at the airport, it would be wise not to proceed to the scene. You do not want to become the next patient. Rushing in to this location could cause you to become a victim, and, as a result, place greater demand on the first response personnel.

■ Question 3

What resources might you call to assist with this situation?

Contacting the EMS dispatcher could lead you to a variety of resources such as local law enforcement, fire departments, hazardous materials units, the FAA (Federal Aviation Administration), and the bomb squad.

■ Question 4

On the basis of the signs and symptoms you were provided, what are the possibilities for the type of agent used?

The signs and symptoms presented here are indicative of nerve agent exposure. The history of nerve agents dates back to World War I, when they were developed to bring mass destruction to opposing forces during war. Terrorist groups are attracted to the use of nerve agents because they have the flexibility of being disseminated in a variety of ways, including release in air, water, or a facility (such as the air ducts of a building). Nerve agents include tabun, sarin, V agent (also known as VX), and soman. They are acutely toxic and have a very rapid effect on the body once exposure has occurred **Table 1**.

Table 1 — The Nerve Agents

Name	Military Designation	Odor	Special Features	Onset of Symptoms	Volatility	Route of Exposure
Tabun	GA	Fruity	Easy to manufacture	Immediate	Low	Contact and vapor hazard
Sarin	GB	None (if pure) or strong	Will off-gas while on victim's clothing	Immediate	High	Primarily respiratory vapor hazard; extremely lethal if skin contact is made
Soman	GD	Fruity	Ages rapidly, making it difficult to treat	Immediate	Moderate	Contact with skin; minimal vapor hazard
V agent	VX	None	Most lethal chemical agent; difficult to decontaminate	Immediate	Very low	Contact with skin; no vapor hazard (unless aerosolized)

Nerve agents can be in gas, aerosol, or liquid form and may enter the body through inhalation or absorption through the skin. They typically have a more rapid onset of signs and symptoms if they are inhaled. This happens because the lungs have a vast supply of blood vessels and the agent can rapidly diffuse across these tissues and get into the circulating blood, thus affecting organs more quickly.

Signs and symptoms found in patients who have been exposed to nerve agents will depend on how the nerve agent has entered the body (inhalation or absorption), as well as the concentration **Table 2**.

Table 2 — Signs and Symptoms of Nerve Agent Exposure

Severity	Symptoms
Mild	• Runny nose • Reduction in pupil size (miosis) • Dimness of vision • Tightness of chest • Difficulty breathing
Moderate	• Increased miosis • Headaches • Confusion • Drowsiness • Nasal congestion • Tightness of chest • Nausea, vomiting, diarrhea • Cramps • Generalized weakness • Twitching of large muscle groups
Severe	• Involuntary defecation and urination • Drooling • Twitching • Staggering • Convulsions • Cessation of breathing • Loss of consciousness • Coma • Death

The onset of signs and symptoms of nerve agents will also depend on dosage and may occur within seconds of exposure to vapors or within minutes to hours of exposure to a liquid form. According to the National Response Center, women tend to be more susceptible to the effects of nerve agents than men.

■ Question 5

What are weapons of mass destruction (WMDs)?

Originally, WMDs were created to maim or kill soldiers in wartime efforts. As the name implies, they are instruments created to bring about a large number of casualties and/or substantial damage to infrastructure and property. WMDs have more recently been used as a terrorist tool to severely injure or kill civilians in many public places. If biological agents (such as anthrax, the plague, or smallpox) are used, the public and responders may not realize it for hours or days later.

■ Question 6

Why are the mnemonics SLUDGEM and DUMBELS used? What does each letter stand for?

These mnemonics are used to describe the signs and symptoms of persons exposed to nerve agents Table 3.

Table 3 Symptoms of Persons Exposed to Nerve Agents

SLUDGEM (military mnemonic)	DUMBELS (medical mnemonic)
Salivation, **S**weating	**D**iarrhea
Lacrimation (excessive tearing)	**U**rination
Urination	**M**iosis (pinpoint pupils)
Defecation, **D**rooling, **D**iarrhea	**B**radycardia, **B**ronchospasm (spasm of the bronchioles)
Gastric upset and cramps	**E**mesis (vomiting)
Emesis (vomiting)	**L**acrimation (excessive tearing)
Muscle twitching/**M**iosis (pinpoint pupils)	**S**eizures, **S**alivation, **S**weating

■ Question 7

What is the EMT's role in a potential terrorism event?

If you are first on scene for a possible terrorist attack, you should take command until another agency is available to do so. Use a reasonable approach to the scene, and do not enter if you suspect a WMD. Take the following precautions until qualified reinforcements arrive:

1. Size up the scene.
2. Provide initial incident command.
3. Notify law enforcement and fire responders.

4. If you are able to do so, do not allow anyone else to enter the location.
5. Back away from the scene to ensure your safety.
6. Avoid parking or staging in a "choke" location (congested area).
7. Identify safe staging areas for incoming responders to use.

It is extremely important to be prepared for a terrorist event, no matter how unlikely it seems. The use of WMDs in our lifetime is a real possibility. EMS, fire agencies, and first response units need to be prepared to recognize and deal with a terrorist event when it happens. Any incident, such as an MCI or WMD incident, will be complex. One definition of an MCI is when the number of patients at a scene overwhelm or exhaust the number of available personnel (such as fire fighters, EMS providers, or police) and available resources.

It is important to understand that MCIs will not always involve WMDs. For example, an MCI may be declared for a traffic collision involving a school bus and a minivan. Some examples of MCIs include plane crashes, tanker truck crashes, building collapses, and apartment fires. These incidents are not intended to be handled by one person or one responding unit. A unified, organized, and cooperative approach is best used when dealing with an MCI or WMD.

For further information on this topic, refer to the *Emergency Response to Terrorism: Job Aid—Edition 2.0*, released by FEMA.

■ Question 8

What are some special considerations when dealing with mass-casualty incidents (MCIs), particularly those that involve a decontamination zone?

Your role as an EMT in an incident involving multiple casualties and decontamination is to report to the command post for further instructions. However, if, as in this scenario, you are first to respond before an MCI has been declared, be sure to identify the event and ask for more resources; then establish a control zone. If the incident does involve a hazardous substance (which could also be a WMD), a specially trained HazMat team will need to be called to the scene to assist in removal of patients from the hot zone (contamination area) through a decontamination zone.

EMTs should not enter the hot zone at any point unless they have been specifically trained as part of a HazMat unit. The patients you receive for treatment should already be decontaminated by the time they get to you. Decontamination involves removing the offending agent or hazardous material from the patient and his or her clothing. Anyone (both personnel and patients) who exits the hot zone *must* be decontaminated prior to receiving any treatment or rehab.

Index

Figures and tables are indicated by *f* and *t* following the page number.

Abdominal massage for obstetric patient, 170
Abdominal pain
   abdominal aortic aneurysm (AAA)
      ALS, working with, 74, 76
      assessment, 72–76, 73t, 74t, 75t, 76t
      case analysis, 77–78
      patient care report, 79
      primary assessment, 72, 73t
      SAMPLE history, 74, 74t
      secondary assessment, 74, 75t
      signs, symptoms, and facts about, 76, 78
      treatment and transport, 74–76
      vital signs, 73t, 75t, 76t
   abdominal evisceration
      ALS, working with, 145, 147, 150
      assessment, 145–146, 145–146t, 147t
      case analysis, 149–150
      mechanism of injury, 146
      patient care report, 151
      primary assessment, 145–146t
      questions to ask, 146, 149
      SAMPLE history, 147t
      secondary assessment, 148t
      treatment and transport, 145, 146, 147, 149, 150
      vital signs, 147t, 149t
   vaginal bleeding, with
      assessment, 100–105, 101t, 102t, 103t, 104t, 105t
      gurney and linens, cleaning, 105, 107
      history questions, additional, 103t, 106
      patient care report, 108
      possible causes, 105–106
      primary assessment, 100–101, 101t
      SAMPLE history, 102t
      secondary assessment, 104t
      transportation, position for, 103, 107
      vital signs, 102t, 105t
Access to patient
   hearing-impaired patient, 192–200, 193t, 194t, 195t, 196t
   motor vehicle extrication and special rescue, 217, 223
Accountability/log-in/log-out rehab sector, 232
Activity (muscle tone) in APGAR scoring system, 173, 173t
Acute myocardial infarction (AMI)
   atypical presentation
      assessment, 53–56, 54t, 55t, 56t, 57t
      case analysis, 57–60, 58t
      most likely patients to have, 60
      patient care report, 61
      primary assessment, 53, 54t
      SAMPLE history, 54–55, 55t
      secondary assessment, 55–57, 56t
      signs and symptoms, 55, 57–58, 58t
      treatment and transport, 56–57
      vital signs, 54t, 57t
   typical presentation signs and symptoms, 58t
Advair Diskus, 49t
Advanced life support (ALS)
   abdominal aortic aneurysm, 74, 76
   abdominal evisceration, 145, 147, 150
   bicyclist struck by motor vehicle, 22, 25
   chest injuries, open, 139, 140
   facial injury, softball pitcher with, 123, 126–127
   fall injury with shock, 38, 40, 43
   lacerations to the forearm, man with, 112, 113
   motor vehicle extrication and special rescue, 220
   neck injury in a swimming pool, 130, 134
   sledding accident, 203
   stroke, 64–65, 69
Airway management
   asthma, 50
   facial injury, softball pitcher with, 123, 125, 127
   management, with CHF, 30, 33
Albuterol, 49t
Allergic reactions, 182
ALS. *See* advanced life support (ALS)
Altered mental status and in police custody, man with
   case analysis, 17–18, 17t, 18t
   patient care report, 19
   primary assessment, 13–15, 14t
   SAMPLE history, 14, 14t
   secondary assessment, 15, 15t
   treatment and transport, 14–16
   vital signs, 15t, 16t
Alupent, 49t
Ambulance collision
   accident statistical overview, 212
   case analysis, 212–214, 214t
   common locations and reasons for, 210, 213
   fatality statistics, 212
   patient care report, 215
   preventive strategies, 211, 213–214
   safe ambulance driving, guidelines for, 211, 214, 214t
   safe driving, factors affecting, 210, 212–213
AMI. *See* acute myocardial infarction (AMI)
APGAR scores, 168t, 169t, 173–174, 173t
Appearance, in APGAR scoring system, 173, 173t
Approach to take
   dog bites, girl with, 116, 119
   facial injury, softball pitcher with, 123, 127
   intoxicated man, 87, 91–92
Arm drift, in Cincinnati Prehospital Stroke Scale, 67t
Aspirin, 56, 59
Assessment, additional
   focused assessment for sledding accident, 203t
   GEMS (Geriatric patients, Environmental assessment, Medical assessment, Social assessment) diamond, 188, 188f
   pediatric assessment triangle, 172, 172f
   rapid trauma assessment, 36–37, 37t
Assistance, additional, determining need for. *See also* advanced life support (ALS)
   illnesses of unknown cause at airport, 236–237, 237f, 239
   lift assist, 3, 5
Asthma
   assessment, 45–48, 46t, 47t, 48t
   case analysis, 49–51, 49f, 49t
   patient care report, 52
   pediatric considerations, 50
   primary assessment, 47t
   respiratory difficulty, 182
   SAMPLE history, 46, 46t
   secondary assessment, 48, 48t
   signs and symptoms, 50
   treatment and transport, 48
   vital signs, 48t
Atrovent, 49t

Back pain and nausea. *See* abdominal pain, abdominal aortic aneurysm (AAA)
Backboards (long boards), uses for, 206t
Bag-mask device
   abdominal aortic aneurysm, 76
   CHF and difficulty breathing, 31, 33
Bariatric patients, lifting, 1–6, 2t, 3t
Basket stretchers (Stokes litters)
   sledding accident, 203, 208
   when to use, 206t
Beclomethasone dipropionate, 49t
Beclovent, 49t
Beconase, 49t
Bicyclist struck by motor vehicle
   case analysis, 24–26
   patient care report, 27
   primary assessment, 20–21, 21t, 24–25
   SAMPLE history, 21–22, 22t, 25
   scene size-up, 20, 24

Bicyclist struck by motor vehicle (cont.)
  secondary assessment, 23t, 26
  vital signs, 21t
Biohazard bags for clean-up
  lacerations to the forearm, 114
  vaginal bleeding, 107
Blankets
  newborns, 167, 169
  sledding accident, 203
  when to use for moving patients, 206t
Bleach solution for clean-up
  lacerations to the forearm, 114
  vaginal bleeding, 107
Blood pressure
  abdominal aortic aneurysm, 73t, 75t, 76t, 77
  fall injury with shock, 35–44, 36t, 37t, 38t, 39t, 40t
  pediatric, normal ranges for, 180t
Blood sugar. See glucose level
Body mechanics for lifting, 5
Breathing difficulty. See also respiratory difficulties
  asthma
    assessment, 45–48, 46t, 47t, 48t
    case analysis, 49–51, 49f, 49t
    patient care report, 52
    primary assessment, 47t
    respiratory difficulty, 182
    SAMPLE history, 46, 46t
    secondary assessment, 48, 48t
    signs and symptoms, 50
    treatment and transport, 48
    vital signs, 48t
  cold symptoms
    assessment, 178–181, 179t, 180t, 181t
    case analysis, 181–182
    patient care report, 183
    primary assessment, 179t
    respiratory difficulties, reasons for, 179, 182
    SAMPLE history, 181t
    scene size-up, 178, 181
    treatment and transport, 179, 181, 182
    vital signs, 180t
  concerns for, with facial injury, 123, 125, 127
  congestive heart failure
    case analysis, 32–33
    patient care report, 34
    primary assessment, 28–29, 29t
    SAMPLE history, 29–30, 30t
    secondary assessment, 31t
    treatment and transport, 30–32
    vital signs, 29t
  COPD
    assessment, 7–9, 8t, 9t
    case analysis, 10–11
    patient care report, 12
    primary assessment, 8, 8t
    SAMPLE history, 8, 9t
    vital signs, 9t
  newborns, concerns for, 169, 172–173, 172f, 173t, 174
Bronchiolitis, 182

Calm situation, ensuring, 22, 25–26
CHART (Chief complaint, History and physical exam, Assessment, R$_x$ (treatment), Transport) format for patient care reports, 17–18, 18t
Chest injuries, open
  ALS, working with, 139, 140
  assessment, 138–140, 139t, 140t, 141t
  case analysis, 142–143
  complications, 139, 143
  legal issues, 142, 143
  patient care report, 144
  primary assessment, 139–140, 139t
  SAMPLE history, 140t
  scene safety, 138, 142
  secondary assessment, 141t
  staging area, 138, 142
  treatment and transport, 139, 140, 142, 143
  vital signs, 140t, 141t
CHF. See congestive heart failure (CHF)
Chronic obstructive pulmonary disease (COPD)
  assessment, 7–9, 8t, 9t
  case analysis, 10–11
  patient care report, 12
  primary assessment, 8, 8t
  SAMPLE history, 8, 9t
  vital signs, 9t
Cincinnati Prehospital Stroke Scale, 64, 64t, 67, 67t
Cleaning the ambulance and equipment
  lacerations to the forearm, 113, 114
  vaginal bleeding, 105, 107
Clothing
  cutting off, for evidence, 142, 143
  motor vehicle extrication and special rescue, 217, 223
Cold packs
  facial injury, 123, 125, 128
  hyperthermia, 161, 165
  leg injuries, 154
Cold symptoms
  assessment, 178–181, 179t, 180t, 181t
  case analysis, 181–182
  patient care report, 183
  primary assessment, 179t
  respiratory difficulties, reasons for, 179, 182
  SAMPLE history, 181t
  scene size-up, 178, 181
  treatment and transport, 179, 181, 182
  vital signs, 180t
Communication
  assisted ventilation, about, 31, 33
  fall injury with shock, 43
  hearing-impaired patient, 192, 193, 196, 197–198
  language barriers, 178, 181
  lift assist, man needing, 4, 5
Compensated shock, 42
Conduction (heat transfer), 163t
Congestive heart failure (CHF)
  case analysis, 32–33
  patient care report, 34
  primary assessment, 28–29, 29t
  SAMPLE history, 29–30, 30t
  secondary assessment, 31t
  treatment and transport, 30–32
  vital signs, 29t
Consent for treatment
  dog bites, girl with, 117, 120
  hip injury, elderly woman with, 184–185, 189
  lacerations to the forearm, teenage girl with, 98
  man with difficulty breathing, 7, 10
Continuous positive airway pressure (CPAP), 33
Convection (heat transfer), 163t
COPD. See chronic obstructive pulmonary disease (COPD)
CPAP (continuous positive airway pressure), 33
Crolom, 49t
Cromolyn sodium, 49t
Croup, 182
Cutivate, 49t

Decontamination areas, 238, 242
Diabetic reactions
  assessment, 80–83, 81t, 82t, 83t
  case analysis, 83–85
  glucose level, checking, 81–82, 84
  patient care report, 86
  primary assessment, 81, 81t
  SAMPLE history, 81, 81t
  treatment, 82
  vital signs, 82t, 83t
Difficulty breathing. See breathing difficulty
Do not resuscitate (DNR) orders, 30
Documentation. See also patient care reports; refusal of treatment and/or transport
  fall by hearing-impaired patient, 196, 199
  fall injury with shock, 43

fire fighter rehab at working fire, 230, 233, 234f
obstetric patient and her newborn, 171, 175
pertinent negatives, 16, 18
SOAP and CHART formats, 17–18, 17t, 18t
Dog bites, girl with
approach to take, 116, 119
assessment, 116–118, 117t, 118t
case analysis, 119–121
dog, concerns about, 117, 120
patient care report, 122
primary assessment, 116, 117t
SAMPLE history, 117–118, 118t
scene size-up, 116, 119
transportation, refusal of, 118–119, 121
treatment, 117, 120
vital signs, 118t
DUMBELS (Diarrhea, Urination, Miosis, Bradycardia, Bronchospasm, Emesis, Lacrimation, Seizures, Salivation, Sweating) symptoms, 238, 241, 241t

Emergency medical technician (EMT) role, working with other emergency responders. *See also* advanced life support (ALS)
motor vehicle extrication and special rescue, 217, 223
potential terrorism event, 238, 241–242
Emergency Response Guidebook (US Department of Transportation), 237, 237f
Emergency vehicle crash. *See* ambulance collision
Emotional support, 134, 136
Epiglottitis, 182
Equipment
leg injuries, 152, 156
moving patients, for, 201, 206, 206t
sledding accident, 201, 206
Evaporation (heat transfer), 163f, 163t
Extrication from motor vehicle and special rescue
accessing the patient, 217, 223
ALS, working with, 220
assessment, 216–220, 218t, 219t, 220t
case analysis, 221–224
extrication process, 218, 223–224
hospital staff, sharing information with, 220, 224
injuries to expect, 216, 221
kinetic energy and severity of injury, 216, 222
MOI, additional history for, 220, 220t
patient care report, 225

primary assessment, 218t
protective clothing to wear, 217, 223
SAMPLE history, 220t
scene size-up, 216–217, 222
secondary assessment, 219
treatment and transport, 218, 220, 223–224
vital signs, 218t, 220t

Facial droop, in Cincinnati Prehospital Stroke Scale, 67t
Facial injury, softball pitcher with
advanced life support, working with, 123, 126–127
approach to take, 123, 127
assessment, 123–126, 124t, 125t, 126t
case analysis, 127–128
mechanism of injury, 123, 127
patient care report, 129
primary assessment, 123, 124t
SAMPLE history, 125, 125t
secondary assessment, 126t
treatment and transport, 123, 125–127
vital signs, 124t
Falls
fall injury with shock
ALS assistance, 38, 40, 43
case analysis, 41–43
patient care report, 44
primary assessment, 36, 36t
rapid trauma assessment, 36–37, 37t
scene size-up, 35, 37
secondary assessment, 39–41, 39t
treatment and transport, 36, 38, 40–41
vital signs, 38t, 40t
hearing-impaired patient, difficult access to
assessment, 192–196, 193t, 194t, 195t, 196t
case analysis, 197–199
communication with patient, 192, 193, 196, 197–198
documentation considerations, 196, 199, 200
hospital staff, sharing information with, 196, 199
patient care report, 200
primary assessment, 193t
SAMPLE history, 193, 194t
scene size-up, 192, 197
secondary assessment, 195t
treatment and transport, 193, 196
vital signs, 194t, 196t
hip injury, elderly woman with
assessment, 184–188, 185t, 186t, 187t
case analysis, 188–189, 188f, 190f
consent for treatment, 184–185, 189

moving the patient to the gurney, 186, 189, 190f
patient care report, 191
primary assessment, 185t
SAMPLE history, 186, 186t
scene size-up, 184, 188, 188f
secondary assessment, 187t
treatment and transport, 186, 187, 189
vital signs, 185t, 186t
leg injuries
assessment, 152–155, 153–154t, 155–156t, 157
case analysis, 156–157
equipment needed, 152, 156
outdoor temperature, 152, 157
patient care report, 158
primary assessment, 153–154t
questions to ask, 153, 157
SAMPLE history, 154t
secondary assessment, 155–156t
treatment and transport, 153–155, 156, 157
vital signs, 154t, 156t
possible reasons for, 198
Fentanyl, 40
Fire fighter rehab at working fire
case analysis, 231–233, 234f
documentation considerations, 230, 233, 234f
emergency incident rehab guidelines, 226, 231
EMS responsibilities, 226, 231–232
fire fighter health and safety, threats to, 227, 232–233
medical conditions to watch for, 227, 233
medical monitoring and assessment, 227, 228, 232, 233
patient care report, 235
primary assessment, 228t
rationale for, 226, 231
rehab sector functions, 226, 232
SAMPLE history, 229, 229t
secondary assessment, 230t
sending fire fighters to rehab, responsibility for, 227, 233
transport to hospital, parameters for, 229
treatment and transport, 227, 229
vital signs, 227t, 228t
Fire hazards
hoarding, 197
oxygen therapy and smoking, 7, 10
Flexible stretchers, use of, 206t
Flonase, 49t
Flovent, 49t
Fluticasone propionate, 49t

Fluticasone propionate and salmeterol xinafoate, 49t
Focused assessment for sledding accident, 203t

Gastric distention, with assisted ventilation, 33
Gastrocom, 49t
Gear/storage area for rehab, 232
GEMS (Geriatric patients, Environmental assessment, Medical assessment, Social assessment) diamond, 188, 188f
Glasgow Coma Scale (GCS), 66, 69–70, 70t
Glucometers, 81–82, 84
Glucose level
　diabetic reaction, 81–82, 84
　low, mimicking stroke, 68
Grimace (irritability), in APGAR scoring system, 173, 173t
Gurneys, use of, 206t

Hazardous materials (HazMat) team, 238
Hearing-impaired patient, difficult access to assessment, 192–196, 193t, 194t, 195t, 196t
　case analysis, 197–199
　communication with patient, 192, 193, 196, 197–198
　documentation considerations, 196, 199, 200
　hospital staff, sharing information with, 196, 199
　patient care report, 200
　primary assessment, 193t
　SAMPLE history, 193, 194t
　scene size-up, 192, 197
　secondary assessment, 195t
　treatment and transport, 193, 196
　vital signs, 194t, 196t
Heart monitors, 140
Heat
　generation of, 162, 163f
　transfer of, 162, 163f, 163t
Heat index, 164f
Heat-related illnesses, populations susceptible to, 161, 162t
Hip injury, elderly woman with
　assessment, 184–188, 185t, 186t, 187t
　case analysis, 188–189, 188f, 190f
　consent for treatment, 184–185, 189
　moving the patient to the gurney, 186, 189, 190f
　patient care report, 191
　primary assessment, 185t
　SAMPLE history, 186, 186t
　scene size-up, 184, 188, 188f
　secondary assessment, 187t
　treatment and transport, 186, 187, 189
　vital signs, 185t, 186t
Histories. See patient history, additional; SAMPLE (Signs/symptoms, Allergies, Medications, Pertinent past medical history, Last oral intake, Events leading up to the injury or illness) history
Hoarding, 192, 197, 199
Hospital staff, sharing information with
　facial injury, softball pitcher with, 127, 128
　fall by hearing-impaired patient, 196, 199
　hyperthermia, 161
　intoxicated man, 90, 92
　motor vehicle extrication and special rescue, 220, 224
　stroke, 66, 68–69, 69t, 70
Hot flashes and nausea. See acute myocardial infarction (AMI)
Humidity and heat index, 164, 164f
Hypertension, 194, 198
Hyperthermia
　assessment, 159–161, 160t, 161t
　case analysis, 161–165, 162t, 163f, 163t, 164f
　hospital staff, sharing information with, 161
　patient care report, 166
　populations most susceptible, 161, 162t
　primary assessment, 160t
　thermoregulation, 162–164, 163f, 163t, 164f
　treatment and transport, 159, 160–161, 165
　vital signs, 161t
　weather, 159, 162–164, 163f, 163t, 164f
Hypothermia
　described and risk factors for, 207
　sledding accident, 207, 207t
　stages of, 207t

Illnesses of unknown cause at airport
　case analysis, 239–242, 240t, 241t
　causes, determination of, 237–238, 237f, 239–241, 240t
　coincidence, determination of, 236, 239
　EMT role in potential terrorism event, 238, 241–242
　nerve agent symptoms, 238, 239–241, 240t, 241t
　resources for assistance, 236–237, 237f, 239
　scene size-up, 236, 239
　special considerations for mass-casualty incidents, 238, 242
　weapons of mass destruction, explained, 238, 241
Inappropriate behavior, accusations of, 98
Infections, respiratory, 182
Injury prevention for EMTs, 3, 4, 5
Intal, 49t
Intoxicated man
　approach to take, 87, 91–92
　assessment, 87–90, 88t, 89t, 90t
　case analysis, 91–92
　patient care report, 93
　primary assessment, 88, 88t
　reliability of history, 88, 92
　SAMPLE history, 88, 89t
　secondary assessment, 90t
　signs and symptoms of intoxication, 87, 91
　transportation, 91
　treatment and transport, 89, 91
　vital signs, 89t
Intravenous (IV) fluids
　abdominal evisceration, 147, 149
　chest injuries, open, 140
　neck injury in a swimming pool, 134
Ipratropium bromide, 49t

Kinetic energy, 216, 222
Knife wounds. See chest injuries, open

Lacerations to the forearm
　man with
　　advanced life support, working with, 112, 113
　　ambulance, cleaning, 113, 114
　　assessment, 109–113, 110t, 111t, 112t, 113t
　　case analysis, 113–114
　　patient care report, 115
　　primary assessment, 109–110, 110t
　　SAMPLE history, 110, 111t
　　secondary assessment, 112t
　　treatment and transport, 110, 111–113, 114
　　vital signs, 111t, 113t
　teenage girl with
　　assessment, 94–97, 95t, 96t
　　case analysis, 97–98, 97t
　　patient care report, 99
　　primary assessment, 94, 95t
　　SAMPLE history, 95, 96t
　　scene safety, 94, 95, 96, 97
　　treatment and transport, 96
　　vital signs, 95t
Language barriers, 178, 181
Leg injuries
　fall from a horse
　　assessment, 152–155, 153–154t, 155–156t, 157

case analysis, 156–157
equipment needed, 152, 156
outdoor temperature, 152, 157
patient care report, 158
primary assessment, 153–154t
questions to ask, 153, 157
SAMPLE history, 154t
secondary assessment, 155–156t
treatment and transport, 153–155, 156, 157
vital signs, 154t, 156t
sledding accident
ALS, working with, 203
assessment, 201–205, 202t, 203t, 204t, 205t
case analysis, 205–208, 206t, 207t
equipment needed, 201, 206
focused assessment, 203t
hypothermia, 207, 207t
moving the patient, 203, 208
patient care report, 209
patient-moving devices, 201, 206, 206t
primary assessment, 202t
SAMPLE history, 205t
scene size-up, 201, 205
secondary assessment, 204t
treatment and transport, 202–205, 207, 207t
vital signs, 203t, 205t
Legal issues. *See also* consent for treatment; documentation; refusal of treatment and/or transport
altered mental status and in police custody, man with, 13–19, 14t, 15t, 16t, 17t, 18t
chest wound, evidence from, 142, 143
lacerations to the forearm, teenage girl with, 96, 98
Level of consciousness
altered mental status and in police custody, man with, 13–16, 14t, 15t
AMI with atypical presentation, 55–56
fall injury with shock, 35, 41
Lift assist, man needing
assessment, 1–2, 2t, 3t
case analysis, 4–5
patient care report, 6
SAMPLE history, 3t
treatment, 2–4
vital signs, 2t, 3t
Limb stabilization
hip injury, elderly woman with, 186, 189
leg injuries, 153, 154, 157
sledding accident, 202
Lip reading, 193, 197
Los Angeles Prehospital Stroke Screen, 67, 68t

Mass and kinetic energy, 216, 222
Mass-casualty incidents. *See* illnesses of unknown cause at airport
Mechanism of injury (MOI)
abdominal evisceration, 146
chest injuries, open, 139
facial injury, softball pitcher with, 123, 127
fall injury with shock, 36, 41
motor vehicle extrication and special rescue, 220, 220t
neck injury in a swimming pool, 131, 135
Meconium stool, 174
Medical evaluation/treatment area for rehab, 232
Medications
administration, six rights of, 51
AMI with atypical presentation, 59
Mental health disorders. *See also* lacerations to the forearm, girl with
evaluation of, 96, 97, 97t
hoarding, 192, 197, 199
Metaprel, 49t
Metaproterenol sulfate, 49t
Metered-dose inhalers, 48, 49, 49f
Minors, consent for treatment of
dog bites, girl with, 117, 120
lacerations to the forearm, teenage girl with, 98
Misting therapy for hyperthermia, 161, 165
MOI. *See* mechanism of injury (MOI)
Motor vehicle crashes
ambulance collision, 210–215, 214t
extrication and special rescue, 216–225, 218t, 219t, 220t
Moving patients
CHF and difficulty breathing, 28, 30, 32
cluttered home, from, 196
extrication from single car MVC, 217, 218, 223–224
hip injury, elderly woman with, 186, 189, 190f
lift assist, technique for, 4, 5
neck injury in a swimming pool, 131, 135
obstetric patient, 167, 172
sledding accident, 203, 208
walking by patients, not allowing, 111, 114
Multisystem trauma from fall injury, 41

Nasalcrom, 49t
Nasopharyngeal airway, 31
Nebulizers, 48, 49
Neck injury in a swimming pool
advanced life support, working with, 130, 134

assessment, 130–134, 132t, 133t, 134t
case analysis, 135–136
emotional support, 134
patient care report, 134, 136, 137
primary assessment, 130–131, 132t
SAMPLE history, 132, 132t
scene size-up, 130, 135
secondary assessment, 133t
treatment and transport, 131, 133, 134, 135
vital signs, 133t, 134t
Nerve agents, exposure to, 239–241, 240t, 241t
Neurologic emergencies
altered mental status and in police custody, man with
case analysis, 17–18, 17t, 18t
patient care report, 19
primary assessment, 13–15, 14t
SAMPLE history, 14, 14t
secondary assessment, 15, 15t
treatment and transport, 14–16
vital signs, 15t, 16t
stroke
advanced life support, working with, 64–65, 69
assessment, 62–66, 63t, 64t, 65t, 66t
case analysis, 67–70, 67t, 68t, 69t, 70t
patient care report, 71
primary assessment, 62, 63t
SAMPLE history, 63–64, 64t
secondary assessment, 65–66, 65t
vital signs, 63t, 66t
Newborns
APGAR scores, 168t, 169t, 173–174, 173t
assessment of, 167–169, 168t, 169t, 171t
assessment tools for, 169, 172–174, 172f, 173f
crying, importance of, 169, 174
patient care report, 177
treatment and transport, 167, 169, 171, 175
Nitroglycerin, 59
Non-verbal communication with hearing-impaired patients, 192, 193, 196, 197–198

Obstetric and neonatal care
ALS, working with, 167
APGAR scores, 168t, 169t, 173–174, 173t
assessment, 167–171, 168t, 169t, 170t, 171t
assessment tools for the newborn, 169, 172–174, 172f, 173t
case analysis, 172–175, 172f, 173t
documentation considerations, 171, 175

Obstetric and neonatal care (cont.)
   patient care reports, 176, 177
   placenta, delivery of, 170
   primary assessment of the mother, 170t
   primary assessment of the newborn, 168t
   questions to ask, 167, 169, 172, 174
   SAMPLE history, 170t
   transportation considerations, 171, 175
   treatment for the mother, 170
   treatment for the newborn, 167, 169
   vital signs for the mother, 171t
   vital signs for the newborn, 168t, 171t
Occlusive dressings for chest wounds, 139, 143
OPQRST (Onset, Provocation/palliation, Quality, Radiation, Severity, Timing) mnemonic for pain, 25
Oral fluid replacement, 227, 229
Oxygen saturation, for AMI with atypical presentation, 59
Oxygen therapy
   abdominal evisceration, 145, 150
   AMI with atypical presentation, 59
   asthma, 48
   CHF and difficulty breathing, 30–31, 32
   cold symptoms, girl with, 179, 182
   facial injury, softball pitcher with, 123
   fall injury with shock, 36
   fire fighter rehab at working fire, 229
   hyperthermia, 159
   lacerations to the forearm, man with, 114
   leg injuries, 153
   neck injury in a swimming pool, 131, 135
   newborns, 169

Pain
   abdominal aortic aneurysm, 74, 76
   facial injury, softball pitcher with, 125, 128
   OPQRST mnemonic, 25
Pain medication
   abdominal evisceration, 147, 149
   fall injury, 40
   sledding accident, 203
Paraplegia, and lifting assistance, 1–6, 2t, 3t
Patient care reports
   abdominal aortic aneurysm, 79
   abdominal evisceration, 151
   abdominal pain and vaginal bleeding, woman with, 108
   access difficulty with hearing-impaired patient, 200
   acute myocardial infarction (AMI) with atypical presentation, 61
   altered mental status in police custody, man with, 19
   ambulance crash, 215
   asthma, girl with, 52
   bicyclist struck by motor vehicle, 27
   chest injuries, open, 144
   CHF and difficulty breathing, 34
   cold symptoms, girl with, 183
   COPD and difficulty breathing, 12
   diabetic reactions, 86
   dog bites, girl with, 122
   facial injury, softball pitcher with, 129
   fall injury with shock, 44
   fire fighter rehab at working fire, 235
   hip injury, elderly woman with, 191
   hyperthermia, 166
   intoxicated man, 93
   lacerations to the forearm, man with, 115
   lacerations to the forearm, teenage girl with, 99
   leg injuries, 158
   lift assist, man needing, 6
   motor vehicle extrication and special rescue, 225
   neck injury in a swimming pool, 134, 136, 137
   newborns, 177
   obstetric patient, 176
   organization of information, 16, 17–18
   sledding accident, 209
   stroke, 71
Patient history, additional. *See also* SAMPLE (Signs/symptoms, Allergies, Medications, Pertinent past medical history, Last oral intake, Events leading up to the injury or illness) history
   abdominal pain and vaginal bleeding, woman with, 103t, 106
   intoxicated man, 88, 92
   motor vehicle extrication and special rescue, 220, 220t
Patient-moving devices, 201, 206, 206t
Pediatric assessment triangle, 172, 172f
Pelvic wrap technique, 42
Pelvis stabilization, 38, 42
Pertinent negatives in documentation, 16, 18
Pertussis (whooping cough), 182
Pets
   dog bites, girl with, 116–122, 117t, 118t
   dogs, securing, 72
   large number of, 192–193, 194, 198–199
Placenta, delivery of, 170
Pneumonia, 182
Poisoning
   nerve agents, exposure to, 239–241, 240t, 241t
   respiratory difficulty, 182
Positioning patients for transport
   abdominal aortic aneurysm, 73, 77
   upright, with difficulty breathing, 28, 32
   woman with abdominal pain and vaginal bleeding, 103, 107
Pressure dressings, 110, 111
Primary assessment
   abdominal aortic aneurysm, 72, 73t
   abdominal pain and vaginal bleeding, woman with, 100–101, 101t
   altered mental status in police custody, man with, 13–15, 14t
   AMI with atypical presentation, 53, 54t
   asthma, 47t
   bicyclist struck by motor vehicle, 20–21, 21t, 24–25
   chest injuries, open, 139–140, 139t
   CHF and difficulty breathing, 28–29, 29t
   cold symptoms, girl with, 179t
   COPD and difficulty breathing, 8, 8t
   diabetic reactions, 81, 81t
   dog bites, girl with, 116, 117t
   facial injury, softball pitcher with, 123, 124t
   fall by hearing-impaired patient, 193t
   fall injury with shock, 36, 36t
   fire fighter rehab at working fire, 228t
   hip injury, elderly woman with, 185t
   hyperthermia, 160t
   intoxicated man, 88, 88t
   lacerations to the forearm, man with, 109–110, 110t
   lacerations to the forearm, teenage girl with, 94, 95t
   leg injuries, 153–154t
   lift assist, man needing, 1, 2t
   motor vehicle extrication and special rescue, 218t
   neck injury in a swimming pool, 130–131, 132t
   newborn, 168t
   obstetric patient, 170t
   sledding accident, 202t
   stroke, 62, 63t
Prioritizing care and transport
   bicyclist struck by motor vehicle, 22, 25
   fall injury with shock, 41–42
   lacerations to the forearm, man with, 110, 113–114
Proventil, 49t
Pulse
   APGAR scoring system, 173, 173t
   pediatric, normal ranges for, 180t

Questions to ask
   abdominal evisceration, 146, 149
   AMI with atypical presentation, 55–56, 58–59
   asthma, girl with, 51
   diabetic reaction, 80, 83

leg injuries, 153, 157
obstetric patients, 167, 169, 172, 174
Qvar, 49t

Radiation (heat transfer), 163t
Rapid trauma assessment, 36–37, 37t
Refusal of treatment and/or transport
  convincing patients to go to the hospital, 55, 58
  diabetic reaction, 82, 84–85
  dog bites, girl with, 118–119, 121
  intoxicated man, 91, 92
  lift assist, man needing, 3
  man with difficulty breathing, 8, 9, 10–11
Respiration
  APGAR scoring system, 173, 173t
  heat transfer, 163t
  pediatric rates, normal ranges for, 180t
Respiratory difficulties. *See also* breathing difficulty
  reasons for, 179, 182
  respiratory failure, signs and symptoms of, 28–29, 32–33
  treatment for, 179, 182
Respiratory syncytial virus (RSV), 182
Rest/refreshment area for rehab, 232

Safety
  chest injuries, open, 138, 142
  cluttered home, 192, 197
  dogs, securing, 72
  fall injury with shock, 35, 41
  lacerations to the forearm, teenage girl with, 94, 95, 96, 97
  lifting bariatric patient, 1–6, 2t, 3t
  man with difficulty breathing, 7, 10
  oxygen therapy and smoking, 7, 10
Salmeterol, 49t
SAMPLE (Signs/symptoms, Allergies, Medications, Pertinent past medical history, Last oral intake, Events leading up to the injury or illness) history
  abdominal aortic aneurysm, 74, 74t
  abdominal evisceration, 147t
  abdominal pain and vaginal bleeding, woman with, 102t
  altered mental status in police custody, man with, 14, 14t
  AMI with atypical presentation, 54–55, 55t
  asthma, 46, 46t
  bicyclist struck by motor vehicle, 21–22, 22t, 25
  chest injuries, open, 140t
  CHF and difficulty breathing, 29–30, 30t
  cold symptoms, girl with, 181t

diabetic reaction, 81, 81t
dog bites, girl with, 117–118, 118t
facial injury, softball pitcher with, 125, 125t
fall by hearing-impaired patient, 193, 194t
fall injury with shock, 37, 38
fire fighter rehab at working fire, 229, 229t
hip injury, elderly woman with, 186, 186t
intoxicated man, 88, 89t
lacerations to the forearm, man with, 110, 111t
lacerations to the forearm, teenage girl with, 95, 96t
leg injuries, 154–155t
lift assist, man needing, 3t
man with difficulty breathing, 8, 9t
motor vehicle extrication and special rescue, 219, 220t
neck injury in a swimming pool, 132, 132t
obstetric patient, 170t
sledding accident, 205t
stroke, 63–64, 64t
Sarin (nerve agent), 239, 240t
Scene size-up
  access difficulty with hearing-impaired patient, 192, 197
  bicyclist struck by motor vehicle, 20, 24
  cold symptoms, girl with, 178, 181
  dog bites, girl with, 116, 119
  fall injury with shock, 35, 37
  hip injury, elderly woman with, 184, 188, 188f
  illnesses of unknown cause at airport, 236, 239
  motor vehicle extrication and special rescue, 216–217, 222
  neck injury in a swimming pool, 130, 135
  sledding accident, 201, 205
Scoop stretchers
  hip injury, 189, 190f
  leg injury, 154
  when to use, 206t
Seat belt use in ambulances, 214, 214t
Secondary assessment
  abdominal aortic aneurysm, 74, 75t
  abdominal evisceration, 148t
  abdominal pain and vaginal bleeding, woman with, 104t
  altered mental status in police custody, man with, 15, 15t
  AMI with atypical presentation, 55–57, 56t
  asthma, 48, 48t

bicyclist struck by motor vehicle, 23t, 26
chest injuries, open, 141t
CHF and difficulty breathing, 31t
facial injury, softball pitcher with, 126t
fall by hearing-impaired patient, 195t
fall injury with shock, 39–41, 39t
fire fighter rehab at working fire, 230t
hip injury, elderly woman with, 187t
intoxicated man, 90t
lacerations to the forearm, man with, 112t
leg injuries, 155–156t
motor vehicle extrication and special rescue, 219t
neck injury in a swimming pool, 133t
sledding accident, 204t
stroke, 65–66, 65t
Serevent, 49t
Sheets for moving patients, 206t
Shock
  abdominal aortic aneurysm, 76, 77
  fall injury, 35–44, 36t, 37t, 38t, 39t, 40t
Short backboards, 206t
Sign language, 196, 198
Six rights of medication administration, 51
Sledding accident
  ALS, working with, 203
  assessment, 201–205, 202t, 203t, 204t, 205t
  case analysis, 205–208, 206t, 207t
  equipment needed, 201, 206
  focused assessment, 203t
  hypothermia, 207, 207t
  moving the patient, 203, 208
  patient care report, 209
  patient-moving devices, 201, 206, 206t
  primary assessment, 202t
  SAMPLE history, 205t
  scene size-up, 201, 205
  secondary assessment, 204t
  treatment and transport, 202–205, 207, 207t
  vital signs, 203t, 205t
SLUDGEM (Salivation, Sweating, Lacrimation, Urination, Defecation, Drooling, Diarrhea, Gastric upset, Emesis, Muscle twitching, Miosis) symptoms, 238, 241, 241t
Small-volume nebulizers, 48, 49
SOAP (Subjective, Objective, Assessment, Plan) format for patient care reports, 17, 17t
Soman (nerve agent), 239, 240t
Speech, in Cincinnati Prehospital Stroke Scale, 67t
Spinal immobilization
  abdominal evisceration, 146

Spinal immobilization (*cont.*)
    altered mental status in police custody, man with, 15
    bicyclist struck by motor vehicle, 22
    chest injuries, open, 139
    facial injury, softball pitcher with, 123, 125
    fall by hearing-impaired patient, 193
    intoxicated man, 89
    motor vehicle extrication and special rescue, 218, 223–224
    neck injury in a swimming pool, 131, 135
Staging area, establishing, 138, 142
Stair chairs
    asthma, 46
    CHF and difficulty breathing, 28, 30, 32
    when to use, 206t
Stokes litters. *See* basket stretchers (Stokes litters)
Stretchers, use of, 206t
Stroke
    advanced life support, working with, 64–65, 69
    assessment, 62–66, 63t, 64t, 65t, 66t
    case analysis, 67–70, 67t, 68t, 69t, 70t
    patient care report, 71
    primary assessment, 62, 63t
    SAMPLE history, 63–64, 64t
    secondary assessment, 65–66, 65t
    vital signs, 63t, 66t
Stroke centers, designation as, 68–69, 69t
Suctioning
    facial injury, softball pitcher with, 125
    newborns, 167, 174

Tabun (nerve agent), 239, 240t
Terrorism response. *See* illnesses of unknown cause at airport
Thermometers, 160, 164
Thermoregulation
    hyperthermia, 162–164, 163f, 163t, 164f
    newborns, 167, 169
Tourniquets, 111, 114
Trainees, sharing information with, 62, 67
Transportation considerations
    fall injury with shock, 42
    obstetric patient and her newborn, 171, 175
    seat belt and restraint use in the ambulance, 214
Tripod position
    asthma, 45
    CHF and difficulty breathing, 28
Twin or multiple births, excluding possibility of, 169

Umbilical cord care with newborns, 167
US Department of Transportation *Emergency Response Guidebook*, 237, 237f

V agent (VX) (nerve agent), 239, 240t
Vaginal bleeding with abdominal pain
    assessment, 100–105, 101t, 102t, 103t, 104t, 105t
    gurney and linens, cleaning, 105, 107
    history questions, additional, 103t, 106
    patient care report, 108
    possible causes, 105–106
    primary assessment, 100–101, 101t
    SAMPLE history, 102t
    secondary assessment, 104t
    transportation, position for, 103, 107
    vital signs, 102t, 105t
Vanceril, 49t
Velocity and kinetic energy, 216, 222
Ventilation, assisted, 31, 32, 33
Ventolin, 49t
Vest-type spinal immobilization
    motor vehicle extrication and special rescue, 223–224
    when to use for moving patients, 206t
Violence, potential for
    forearm lacerations, teenage girl with, 95, 97
    knife wound to the chest, 138, 142
Vital sign monitoring/determination rehab sector, 232
Vital signs, baseline
    abdominal aortic aneurysm, 73t
    abdominal evisceration, 147t
    abdominal pain and vaginal bleeding, woman with, 102t
    altered mental status in police custody, man with, 15t
    AMI with atypical presentation, 54t
    asthma, 48t
    bicyclist struck by motor vehicle, 21t
    chest injuries, open, 140t
    CHF and difficulty breathing, 29t
    cold symptoms, girl with, 180t
    diabetic reaction, 82t
    dog bites, girl with, 117t
    facial injury, softball pitcher with, 124t
    fall by hearing-impaired patient, 194t
    fall injury with shock, 38t
    fire fighter rehab at working fire, 227t
    hip injury, elderly woman with, 185t
    hyperthermia, 161t
    intoxicated man, 89t
    lacerations to the forearm, man with, 111t
    lacerations to the forearm, teenage girl with, 95t
    leg injuries, 154t
    lift assist, man needing, 2t
    man with difficulty breathing, 9t
    motor vehicle extrication and special rescue, 218t
    neck injury in a swimming pool, 133t
    newborn, 168t
    obstetric patient, 171t
    sledding accident, 203t
    stroke, 63t
Vital signs, pediatric, normal ranges for, 180t
Vital signs, subsequent
    abdominal aortic aneurysm, 75t, 76t
    abdominal evisceration, 149t
    abdominal pain and vaginal bleeding, woman with, 105t
    altered mental status in police custody, man with, 16t
    AMI with atypical presentation, 57t
    chest injuries, open, 141t
    cold symptoms, girl with, 180t
    diabetic reaction, 83t
    fall by hearing-impaired patient, 196t
    fall injury with shock, 40t
    fire fighter rehab at working fire, 228t
    hip injury, elderly woman with, 186t
    intoxicated man, 89t
    lacerations to the forearm, man with, 113t
    leg injuries, 156t
    lift assist, man needing, 3t
    motor vehicle extrication and special rescue, 220t
    neck injury in a swimming pool, 134t
    newborn, 171t
    sledding accident, 205t
    stroke, 66t
Volmax, 49t

Walking by patients, not allowing, 111, 114
Weapons of mass destruction (WMDs), described, 238, 241
Weather
    asthma, 45
    cold temperature, and leg injuries, 152, 157
    fall injury with shock, 35, 37
    hot, and hyperthermia, 159, 162–164, 163f, 163t, 164f
Whooping cough (pertussis), 182
Wound care
    abdominal evisceration, 146, 147, 150
    chest injuries, open, 139, 143
    dog bites, girl with, 117, 120
    fall injury with shock, 40, 42
    lacerations to the forearm, man with, 110, 111

Photo Credits

Case Study Openers
© Michael Ledray/ShutterStock, Inc.

Case Study 7
Figure 1 © Photos.com

Case Study 22
Figure 2 Courtesy of the National Weather Service.

Case Study 23
Figure 1 Courtesy of the American Academy of Pediatrics

Case Study 31
Figure 1 Courtesy of the U.S. Department of Transportation.

Unless otherwise indicated, all photographs and illustrations are under copyright of Jones & Bartlett Learning.

Some images in this book feature models. These models do not necessarily endorse, represent, or participate in the activities represented in the images.